THE RESPIRATORY FUNCTION
OF THE BLOOD

PART II
HÆMOGLOBIN

THE RESPIRATORY FUNCTION
OF THE BLOOD

PART II

HÆMOGLOBIN

by

JOSEPH BARCROFT

Fellow of King's College, Cambridge

CAMBRIDGE

AT THE UNIVERSITY PRESS

1928

CAMBRIDGE
UNIVERSITY PRESS

University Printing House, Cambridge CB2 8BS, United Kingdom

Published in the United States of America by Cambridge University Press, New York

Cambridge University Press is part of the University of Cambridge.

It furthers the University's mission by disseminating knowledge in the pursuit of
education, learning and research at the highest international levels of excellence.

www.cambridge.org
Information on this title: www.cambridge.org/9781107415881

First published 1928
First paperback edition 2014

A catalogue record for this publication is available from the British Library

ISBN 978-1-107-41588-1 Paperback

....

PREFACE

TO THE FIRST EDITION OF

THE RESPIRATORY FUNCTION OF THE BLOOD

At one time, which seems too long ago, most of my leisure was spent in boats. In them I learned what little I know of research, not of technique or of physiology, but of the qualities essential to those who would venture beyond the visible horizon.

The story of my physiological "ventures" will be found in the following pages. Sometimes I have sailed single handed, sometimes I have been one of a crew, sometimes I have sent the ship's boat on some expedition without me. Any merit which attaches to my narrative lies in the fact that it is in some sense at first hand. I have refrained from discussing subjects which I have not actually touched, but which might fittingly have been included in a modern account of the blood as a vehicle for oxygen. Such are the relation of narcosis to oxygen-want and the properties of intracellular oxidative enzymes. The omission of these and other important subjects has made the choice of a title somewhat difficult. I should like to have called the book, what it frankly is—a log; did not such a title involve an air of flippancy quite out of place in the description of the serious work of a man's life. I have therefore chosen a less exact, though more comprehensive title.

After all, the pleasantest memories of a cruise are those of the men with whom one has sailed. The debt which I owe to my colleagues, whether older or younger than myself, will be evident enough to any reader of the book. It leaves me well-nigh bankrupt—a condition well known to most sailors. But I owe another large debt of gratitude to those who, as teachers, showed me the fascination of physiology, to Dr Kimmins *, and especially to

* Formerly science master of the Leys School, now Chief Inspector of the Educational Department of the London County Council.

Dr Anderson*. At a later stage I learned much from Dr Gaskell, Professor Langley and Dr Haldane.

There are occasions on which every sailor of the deep sea has to ship a pilot. Mr A. V. Hill has brought me into those harbours which are best approached through the, to me, unknown channels of mathematics.

* Formerly supervisor in physiology to King's College, now Master of Gonville and Caius College.

J. B.

CAMBRIDGE,
December, 1913.

PREFACE TO HÆMOGLOBIN

THE rapid advance of knowledge rendered impossible the task of revising *The Respiratory Function of the Blood* for a second edition. The book was in three parts with an Appendix on technique: there is now more than enough known about the subject-matter of each part to justify a book on that alone. I have therefore determined to break up the volume into a *series* of manageable units, originally intended to correspond more or less to the "Parts" of the original work. The first volume of this series, *Lessons from High Altitudes*, appeared in 1925, the second is now presented.

The present volume deals with hæmoglobin regarded as a chemical substance; and here I would like particularly to point to the limited scope of this book. It makes no profession of dealing with the red blood corpuscle, or with the properties of blood. These will form the subject of another volume. Thus the consideration of many now classical investigations, such as those of the Rockefeller Institute and the nomogram of Prof. L. J. Henderson, is reserved for the present.

I have to thank the Royal Society for permission to reproduce Figs. 2, 6, 7, 14, 28, 33, 40, 41, 42, 43, 44, 45, 46 A and B; the Chemical Society for Figs. 15 and 16; the American Chemical Society for Fig. 17; the Editors of *The Journal of Biological Chemistry* for Figs. 34 and 38 and *The Journal of Physiology* for Figs. 8, 9, 10, 29, 30 and 59. For allowing me to reproduce their figures and for much help at various stages my thanks are due to Dr H. Hartridge, Dr D. Keilin, Dr F. J. W. Roughton, Mr G. S. Adair and Mr R. Hill: indeed if the work has any merit it will be largely due to their efforts. For assistance with the proofs and the bibliography I am much indebted to Mrs Thacker, late Fellow of Newnham College and to Miss N. Henderson.

My debt would not be discharged without one more reference. The expense of much of the later phases of the work done on hæmoglobin in this country has been borne by the Medical Research Council—a department of the Privy Council. How that body came to act "in loco parentis" is worth placing on record. Readers of the book will find that the late Sir William Bayliss was sceptical about the interpretation of much that had been written on hæmoglobin; on the initiative of Prof. A. V. Hill an invitation was sent to him to come to Cambridge and sift the points at issue so far as that could be done by discussion. Many points seemed capable of experimental proof or disproof and Bayliss conceived the idea of interesting the Department of Scientific and Industrial Research in hæmoglobin. The subject fell rather within the sphere of the Medical Research Council who took the matter up and have assisted hæmoglobin research both with funds, sympathy and advice ever since. In thanking the Committee I feel that I must also thank the secretary, Sir Walter Morley Fletcher.

J. B.

CAMBRIDGE,
3 *April*, 1928.

CONTENTS

CHAPTER I

INTRODUCTORY

Sir michael foster(1) likened the growth of knowledge to the ascent of a spiral stair from which the observer periodically surveys the same landscape, but each time from a higher level than the last. In the decade before the war great advances were made in an understanding of hæmoglobin, and even then sufficient was known about it to elicit, if not to justify, the statement (2) that hæmoglobin "was perhaps the second most interesting substance in the world"—the first presumably being chlorophyll. The landscape spread out before the observer then was that of hæmoglobin behaving differently under all sorts of circumstances. The point of view on the spiral which was attained was the discovery that circumstances themselves had a quite unexpectedly great effect in regulating the action of hæmoglobin, so that the question was seriously asked whether all hæmoglobin was not really the same. The answer at one time appeared almost to be "yes." Those whose philosophy ran in the direction of a single hæmoglobin, had still to face the fact that the pigment from the corpuscles of different animals crystallised differently (3). That, in 1910, seemed a small matter as compared with the divergences which had been shown merely to be a matter of circumstance—solvent, temperature, hydrogen-ion concentration and the like. With an understanding of the necessity for the study of hæmoglobin under uniform conditions the whole question of the uniformity of hæmoglobin was ripe for reinvestigation. A few experiments made on the subject by Douglas, Haldane and Haldane (4) before the war pointed to the existence of essential differences in the hæmoglobin of different species.

Since 1921 the whole matter has been gone into in great detail, and to-day we are confronted with the same landscape, which ten years previously appeared to consist merely of a few massive features: from our present height it consists of endless detail.

Both abroad (Vlès (5)) and at home (6) it was shown that the hæmoglobin of *Arenicola* differed essentially from that of man, both spectroscopically and in its gas-binding properties. The discovery of this difference led to a systematic comparison of the hæmoglobins of many forms of life[7]. Of these one of the most fruitful was the comparison between the hæmoglobin in the larva of the fly *Gastrophilus* and that of the horse[7], [8], the point of the comparison being that the *Gastrophilus* larva grows in the equine stomach. But though the larval hæmoglobin is manufactured in the horse it is not the same spectroscopically as the horse's hæmoglobin. Moreover it is not evident why the *Gastrophilus* larva should contain hæmoglobin at all. The primary use of hæmoglobin in the Mammalia is for oxygen transport. In *Gastrophilus* larva the hæmoglobin is fixed and the same is true of the hæmoglobin in mammalian muscles and many other places. Keilin therefore was led into an investigation of the structure and function of hæmoglobin in muscle—this research led to his discovery of cytochrome[8], a body closely related to hæmoglobin, which is very widely distributed throughout the animal and vegetable kingdoms—so much so as to challenge the question whether it or its constituents are not really more primitive than chlorophyll.

What is the nature of the differences between one hæmoglobin and another?

Clearly there is the possibility that as between two different samples of hæmoglobin, the hæmatin may be uniform and the globin may differ. Or the globin may be the same and the hæmatin may differ. Or both the globins and the hæmatins may differ.

One method of attacking the question was to treat the hæmoglobin with alkali in the presence of a reducing agent. The idea—erroneous as it turned out—was that the globin would be split from the hæmatin and the resulting spectrum would be that of reduced hæmatin in alkaline solution. In this task Anson and Mirsky[9] repeated (though quite independently) an observation which had appeared sporadically in the previous literature but the importance of which had never been appreciated (Bertin-Sans and Moitessier[10], and Dilling[11]), namely, that hæmochromogen is not reduced hæmatin in alkaline solution, but is a compound of that body with globin. Anson and Mirsky[9], working over a number of mammalian bloods, found that the spectra of the hæmochromogens which they yielded were identical. From this it may be gathered that in this range of hæmoglobins the hæmatin portion is identical in all, and that the globins are different.

The question arises then: If the globins are different in the hæmoglobins of the horse and the mouse, why have the hæmochromogens identical spectra? That question leads to another: What is the essential difference between hæmoglobin and hæmochromogen? Anson and Mirsky [9] answer this question as follows: Hæmoglobin is hæmatin united with undenatured globin—hæmochromogen is united with denatured protein.

The differences in the globin moiety only carry us a certain way. There are certainly hæmoglobins which differ in the hæmatin moiety —hæmatin is essentially a compound of iron with porphyrin, and porphyrin is essentially a compound containing four pyrrol groupings. As there can be many porphyrins, according as the side chains differ slightly, so conceivably there can be as many hæmoglobins. Three such have been prepared by Hill and Holden [12], they are the hæmo-globins which correspond to proto-, meso- and hæmatoporphyrins. There is also one such body which has not been prepared synthetically but which was found in the blood of certain polychæte worms by Ray Lankester [13] and the true nature of which has recently been recognised by Fox [14].

Porphyrins may unite with metals other than iron, as has been shown by numerous observers (Laidlaw [15], Schulz [16], Milroy [17]). Knowledge of the metalloporphyrins has been much extended by R. Hill [18], but though he has made many attempts to prepare hæmoglobins from metalloporphyrins containing metals other than iron, these have been unsuccessful. Globin will not unite with them: and from the other side, though hæmochromogens may be pre-pared by the addition of many substances (hydrazine, nicotine, pyridine) to hæmatin, globin is the only such material which by its association with oxygen yields a body from which the oxygen is detachable by mere exposure to a vacuum.

Hæmochromogen forms no reversible oxide. Attempts to oxidise it in alkaline solution appear to break it down. An oxide in neutral solution is stable, but it cannot be reduced by a vacuum. It has been studied by Keilin [19] and is called by him "parahæmatin" (formerly it was known as kathæmoglobin). While oxygen does not unite reversibly with hæmochromogen, carbon monoxide does. It is possible to determine the curve, as was done by Anson and Mirsky [9], which expresses the equilibrium between CO and hæmochromogen. Revert-ing from hæmochromogen to hæmoglobin, the affinity of CO for the pigment is about 400 times that of oxygen in man, and perhaps 100 times that of oxygen in the rabbit—the relative affinities of the two gases differing for the hæmoglobins of different animals.

To the great affinity of CO for hæmoglobin, has been attributed

its danger as a poison, the current view being that CO itself is in-
nocuous, but that uniting with the hæmoglobin of the body it prevents
the carriage of the oxygen, necessary for life, to the brain and other
organs. It might be inferred that to forms of life which did not depend
on hæmoglobin for their oxygen supply, carbon monoxide would
be harmless. Yet this is not the case. Warburg[20] has shown that CO
inhibits the oxygen uptake of yeast and J. B. S. Haldane[21] that both
to growing seedlings and to moths carbon monoxide is poisonous even
though these forms of life are devoid of hæmoglobin. Moreover,
the poisonous dose does not depend upon the absolute amount of
carbon monoxide present but on its concentration relative to that
of oxygen.

The union of carbon monoxide in such small concentrations with
hæmoglobin has been analysed by Hartridge and Roughton[22]. The
equilibrium constant of each of the reactions

$$CO + Hb \rightleftarrows COHb$$

and

$$O_2 + Hb \rightleftarrows O_2Hb$$

is of course the quotient of the velocity constants of the two phases
of the reaction. Hartridge and Roughton, by extraordinarily ingenious methods, have measured the four velocity constants involved,
and found that the great affinity of CO for hæmoglobin is due not to
the great magnitude of the velocity constant for the phase

$$CO + Hb \longrightarrow COHb,$$

but to the small value of the constant for

$$CO + Hb \longleftarrow COHb.$$

The equation

$$CO + Hb = COHb,$$

written in that way, expresses a heritage of convention, for the
molecular weight of hæmoglobin has at last been determined in
two quite different ways independently by two observers. By a
curious irony one of these methods depends upon its extreme slowness,
the other on its extreme speed. Adair[23], by measurements of the
osmotic pressure, each measurement extending over months, has
found the osmotic pressure over a great range of conditions to correspond to about 70,000. This figure is the same as that more recently
obtained by Svedberg[24], who, spinning solutions of hæmoglobin
at about 10,000 revolutions per minute, actually concentrated the

hæmoglobin molecules in the peripheral portion, with sufficient precision to calculate the molecular weight. The molecular weight of 70,000 or thereabouts introduces fresh possibilities as to the differences between one form of hæmoglobin and another. The molecular weight which would correspond to an atom of iron is about 17,000, or approximately one-quarter of the true molecular weight. We do not know how the hæmatin is attached to the globin, but it would appear either that four hæmatins are attached to one globin, or four molecules, each of 17,000 molecular weight, are condensed. In either case the process might admit of great variations in detail. The establishment of the fourfold molecular weight leaves us with some difficulties:

(1) In its relation to oxygen hæmoglobin reacts very much as though one molecule of oxygen united with one of hæmoglobin. Hartridge and Roughton[25] suggest that possibly in this very large molecule the four hæmatins may be so far apart as each to unite with oxygen as though the others were non-existent.

(2) Hæmoglobin in its relations with oxygen behaves also as though in solution. This is true whether in ordinary aqueous solution or in the red blood corpuscles. Yet the red blood corpuscles of many animals, if hæmolysed even under the most rigorous conditions and without either concentration or dilution of the hæmoglobin, shed it as crystalline material. Why should the mere breaking of the structure of a cell throw the material within it out of solution? Presumably in the cell the molecules are not free to orientate themselves at pleasure. The direction of their orientation is in some way decided by the structure of the cell and the whole of the biological aspect is regulated by that orientation. If that be true of the hæmoglobin in the red corpuscle, of how many other substances and in how many other cells may it not also be true?

REFERENCES

(1) FOSTER. In an unpublished lecture.

(2) HENDERSON, L. J. In conversation.

(3) The literature is given in the exhaustive treatise, *The Crystallography of Hæmoglobins*, by REICHERT AND BROWN. 1909.

(4) DOUGLAS, HALDANE AND HALDANE. *Journ. Physiol.* XLIV. 275. 1912.

(5) VLÈS. *Arch. de Phys. Biol.* II. 22. 1922.

(6) BARCROFT, J. AND BARCROFT, H. *Proc. Roy. Soc.* B. XCVI. 28. 1924.

(7) ANSON, BARCROFT, MIRSKY AND OINUMA. *Proc. Roy. Soc.* B. XCVII. 61. 1925.

(8) KEILIN. *Proc. Roy. Soc.* B. XCVIII. 312. 1925; C. 129. 1926.

(9) ANSON AND MIRSKY. *Journ. Physiol.* LX. 50. 1925.

(10) BERTIN-SANS AND MOITESSIER. *C. R. Ac. Sci. Paris*, CXVI. 591. 1893.

(11) DILLING. *Atlas of Hæmochromogens.* Stuttgart, 1910. *Atlas der Krystallformen u. Absorptionbänder der Hämochromogene.*

(12) HILL AND HOLDEN. *Biochem. Journ.* XX. 1326. 1926.

(13) LANKESTER, E. RAY. *Journ. Anat. and Physiol.* II. 114 (1867); III. 119. (1870).

(14) FOX. *Proc. Roy. Soc.* B. XCIX. 199. 1926.

(15) LAIDLAW. *Journ. Physiol.* XXXI. 464. 1904.

(16) SCHULZ. *Arch. f. Anat. u. Physiol.* Suppl. 271. 1904.

(17) MILROY. *Journ. Physiol.* XXXVIII. 384. 1909.

(18) HILL, R. *Biochem. Journ.* XIX. 341. 1925.

(19) KEILIN. *Proc. Roy. Soc.* B. C. 129. 1926.

(20) WARBURG. *Bioch. Zeitsch.* CLXXVII. 471. 1926.

(21) HALDANE, J. B. S. *Nature*, CXIX. 352. 1927.

(22) HARTRIDGE AND ROUGHTON. Communication to the Physiol. Soc. June 1926.

(23) ADAIR. *Proc. Roy. Soc.* A. CVIII. 627. 1925; CIX. 292. 1925.

—— Abstract of Communication to XIIth Internat. Physiol. Congress at Stockholm. *Skand. Archiv.* 1926.

—— "The Application of Dalton's Law of Partial Pressures in the Interpretation of the O.P. of Proteins." And, "The Activity Coefficients of Protein ions." *Trans. Farad. Soc.* Ap. 1927. (In Press.)

(24) SVEDBERG AND FÅHRENS. *Journ. Am. Chem. Soc.* XLVIII. 430. 1926. Also SVEDBERG AND LYSHOLM. *Nova Acta regiae societatis scientiarum Upsaliensis.* Volumen extra ordinem, 1927.

(25) HARTRIDGE AND ROUGHTON. *Proc. Roy. Soc.* A. CVII. 654. 1925.

CHAPTER II

PORPHYRINS

THERE are stories in Cambridge which go back to the days in which Michael Foster sowed such seed as grew up to form the English school of modern physiology. One of these stories has to do with his pupil, Francis Maitland Balfour, the embryologist. It is related (with what truth I cannot say) that Balfour as a young man asked Foster to suggest to him a subject for research. Foster was taking lunch at the time and before him was a boiled egg. He pointed to the egg and said, "What better subject can you have than that?" And there the study of hæmoglobin may commence also; for the particular material which at the moment is regarded as the material starting-point in hæmoglobinology is porphyrin, the brown colouring matter of many eggs. I say "at the moment" because twenty years ago, or even less, the study of hæmoglobin was supposed to have its source in chlorophyll; but the most competent judges, for instance Willstätter(1), regard it as difficult to attach evolutional significance to the chemical similarity between chlorophyll and porphyrin. Even though the view that hæmoglobin in the animal kingdom is the direct result of chlorophyll which is eaten in vegetable food has found recent supporters in Verne (2) and Marchelewski(3), it seems not proven. Let us commence then with porphyrin as being the simplest pigment which has evident chemical relationships with hæmoglobin.

Porphyrin, apart from its existence in the egg-shell, does not bulk very large in warm-blooded animals, though in small quantities it is widely distributed. In the earthworm it constitutes the line of pigment down the back and is found in many other places in invertebrates (MacMunn, Dhéré, Derrien). To distinguish it from the other members of its class (which comprises other natural porphyrins such as uro- and coproporphyrin) it is known as Kämmerer's porphyrin. More recently it has been called by Hans Fischer (4) (who has crowned a compendious series of researches by synthesising some members of the porphyrin group) protoporphyrin. The names ooporphyrin and Kämmerer's porphyrin are significant, for they serve to remind the reader that the material found in the egg-shell is the same as that obtained from blood by Kämmerer. He produced this substance as a degradation product of hæmoglobin by the action on it of

certain bacteria, and so, naturally, the question arises: What is the
relation between ooporphyrin and the simplest crystalline product
of the hæmatin family—hæmin for instance? So far as their empirical formulæ are concerned the relationship would be as follows:

$$\begin{array}{ll}
\text{Ooporphyrin} & C_{34}H_{30}N_4O_4 \cdot H_2 \\
\text{Hæmin} & C_{34}H_{30}N_4O_4FeCl \\
\text{Hæmatin} & C_{34}H_{30}N_4O_4FeOH.
\end{array}$$

Here let me make a short digression to point out the essential nature
of these formulæ. Written as graphic formulæ they, at first sight,
look almost as alarming as the modern "cross-word puzzle." Yet a
moment's consideration will show that in their main features they
are easily grasped.

The fundamental grouping of atoms on which the whole pivots is
the pyrrol ring, consisting of four carbon atoms and one nitrogen
atom joined together in the form of a five-pointed figure

pyrrol itself being

The above is written in an abbreviated form

It is when two such rings are joined together in the following way
that the molecule takes on the first vestige of porphyrin character:

Let us double once more and we obtain[1]

(Hans Fischer.)

This is clearly the skeleton, so to speak, to which the soft parts in the way of side chains are attached. On this skeleton are built up not only all the porphyrins but so far as is known all vertebrate blood pigments.

Let us fill in the "soft parts."

This probably represents the brown pigment of the egg-shell: its relation to the blood pigments is a matter of exchanging for two hydrogens the group FeOH thus:

which is hæmatin, or by FeCl which gives hæmin.

---

[1] Kuster had published an alternative linkage of the four pyrrols which Fischer, since the above went to press, has adopted. [*Berichte Jahrg.* LX. Seite 2611, 1927.]

To return from the digression on the pyrrol structure of porphyrin, I had pointed out that the essential difference between hæmatin and ooporphyrin was the replacement of the FeOH group of the hæmatin by two hydrogen atoms, and further I had said that the replacement could be effected by the action of certain bacteria, at all events when blood was used as the starting-point. The usual method, however, of removing the iron from hæmin is by the action of strong sulphuric acid, or better by hydrobromic acid; in that case the FeCl is replaced not merely by two hydrogen atoms, but two molecules of water are added at the same time. The substance is not ooporphyrin but hæmatoporphyrin, $C_{34}H_{38}N_4O_6$. The hydration takes place in the two groupings indicated below:

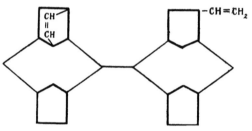

Put in two molecules of water H.OH and you might get:

but equally if the water went in to the same groupings in another way, the following might be obtained:

And there are six other ways in which the two water molecules might be included on similar lines. Each of the bodies so formed is not only a porphyrin but a hæmatoporphyrin. So that there are eight slightly different bodies all of which are obtained by the hydration of two groupings in the protoporphyrin (ooporphyrin) and are isomeric forms of hæmatoporphyrin.

In point of fact hæmatoporphyrin, as we know it, is probably a mixture of the whole eight substances, each of which differs so slightly from its fellows as to be scarcely distinguishable as a separate unit. But there are other porphyrins, coproporphyrin for instance which has the formula

and uroporphyrin

Two questions naturally arise: (1) Is it possible to make hæmoglobins corresponding to porphyrins other than protoporphyrin? and (2) Do any such forms of hæmoglobin occur in nature?

Both these questions can be answered in the affirmative. Hill and Holden(5), working in the Cambridge Biochemical Laboratory, have succeeded in preparing hæmoglobins corresponding to hæmatoporphyrin and mesoporphyrin—a process which involves not merely the production of the oxyhæmoglobin itself but on the way the corresponding hæmin, methæmoglobin and reduced hæmoglobin. Thus there is no reason why nature should not abound with countless forms of hæmoglobin each differing from its neighbour by some trifling dissimilarity in the structure of its specific porphyrin. Hitherto only one form of hæmoglobin has been found in nature which has a porphyrin basis other than that of protoporphyrin. That hæmoglobin occurs very far down in the animal kingdom (in some polychæte worms) and for a reason which we do not know nature seems not to have persisted in it. It is called chlorocruorin.

Chlorocruorin is, if I may say so, an old love of Ray Lankester's(6); he first described it and, as I know by talking with him, he has never lost interest in it and in the discovery of its relation to hæmoglobin. Green in dilute solution, chlorocruorin is reddish when more concentrated. Lankester showed that it could be oxidised and reduced as hæmoglobin could be, and that like hæmoglobin the oxy-body had two absorption bands in the visible spectrum whilst the reduced body had but one. The bands of chlorocruorin, whilst similar to those of hæmoglobin, are not identical with the hæmoglobin bands in position. They are nearer the red end of the spectrum, not by a little but by a great deal. The β-band of chlorocruorin (that nearest the blue end of the spectrum) occupies a position about half-way between the α- and β-bands of hæmoglobin, whilst the α-band of chlorocruorin is displaced correspondingly towards the red. The actual difference in the positions of maximum density of the α-bands of chlorocruorin and of hæmoglobin is of the order of 250–300 Ångström units. So great a difference is not surprising in the light of the work of Hill and Holden, for the hæmoglobins (and their derivatives) prepared from meso- and from hæmatoporphyrins had spectra of the same general character as those of the corresponding compounds of ordinary hæmoglobin, but considerably displaced towards the blue end. The spectrum of hæmoglobin therefore occupies a position intermediate between that of chlorocruorin and those of the hæmoglobins made from meso- and hæmatoporphyrins. It is to H. Munro Fox(7) that we owe our recent knowledge of chlorocruorin. He it was who solved the problem so near to Lankester's heart—the relation of that body to hæmoglobin. Fox showed that there was in addition to the oxy-body, the reduced body and the body analogous to hæmochromogen, a complete series of hæmoglobin analogues. Moreover—and this is the point that matters—the difference between the hæmoglobin bodies and the chlorocruorin bodies is that the latter are built up on a different foundation of porphyrin from the former. Whereas all forms of hæmoglobin hitherto found in nature are derivatives of protoporphyrin, chlorocruorin is a derivative of some other and as yet unknown member of the porphyrin series.

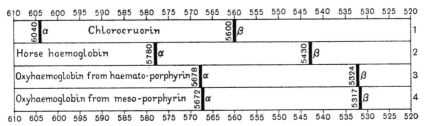

Fig. 1. (1) Position of α- and β-bands of chlorocruorin (Fox). (2) Position of α- and β-bands of horse hæmoglobin (Fox). (3) Position of α- and β-bands of oxyhæmoglobin made from hæmatoporphyrin (Hill and Holden). (4) Position of α- and β-bands of oxyhæmoglobin made from mesoporphyrin (Hill and Holden).

At this point I can claim to become a little reminiscent, for the mention of strong sulphuric acid coupled with hæmatoporphyrin carries me back in memory to the "old physiological laboratory," the same in which Foster fired Balfour with a zeal for embryology; to the room, on the opposite side of the passage from Foster's, in which Hopkins isolated tryptophane and in which Laidlaw, under his benign influence, made the following observation, namely, that whilst the strongest possible reagents, such as concentrated H_2SO_4, are required for the dislodgement of the iron from oxyhæmoglobin, only very weak acid is necessary for the formation of porphyrin from reduced hæmoglobin. In the case of Laidlaw's original observation the blood was reduced by bacterial action, but he showed that there was nothing specific about that; any form of reduction would serve. For the moment I will pass over the great significance of Laidlaw's observation as showing the intimate connection between the lability of iron in hæmoglobin and the oxygen and proceed directly to three other observations of Laidlaw's [8] which are in the straight line of our present enquiry: (1) that he could put back the iron and so build up hæmatin from porphyrin[1]; (2) that he could, instead of putting in iron, put in cobalt, thus indicating the possibility of producing a whole series of compounds of porphyrin with different metals; and (3) that by uniting porphyrin with copper he produced a substance which seemed to be, but was not quite identical with the pigment turacin which is extracted from the feathers of the South African bird *Turaco*. This pigment has always evoked a mild interest because, being somewhat soluble in dilute alkali, it disappears from the feathers during the rainy season. The nest is contaminated with the alkaline excrement of the bird; and the excrement becoming moistened by the rain dissolves the turacin.

Laidlaw, then, extended the field of interest in porphyrin, on the chemical side, by showing that the iron-porphyrin compound was only one of a number of "metalloporphyrins" and, on the biological side, by showing that the copper porphyrin was responsible for a pigment of very different biological significance from hæmoglobin.

In both fields, that of the metalloporphyrins and that of turacin, great advances have been made within recent years.

With regard to metalloporphyrins Schulz[9] in 1904 (the same year in which Laidlaw prepared the copper and cobalt porphyrins) made the zinc body, Milroy[10] in 1909 manufactured a nickel and a tin metalloporphyrin, and now the compounds with aluminium silver, sodium and potassium have all been carefully studied by Robert Hill[11]. Of these only three can be oxidised and reduced, namely the compounds of cobalt (as shown by Laidlaw), iron and manganese.

To pass to turacin, which was first described by Church[12]. A few lines back I said that the turacin of the feathers was *dissolved* by dilute alkali: that statement needs some justification. It is true that when the feathers are treated with alkali pigment leaves the feathers and appears in the alkali. But is the process merely one of solution? or is the turacin changed into something else? The reason for suspicion is that the spectrum of the pigment observed in the alkali differs from that seen in the feathers. What then are these spectra, and how are they related? These matters have been studied by Keilin[13] and are of great importance on account of the light which they throw upon the constitution of pigments of much wider distribution than turacin.

---

[1] The difference between the different porphyrins was not recognised at the time of Laidlaw's work, actually it was ooporphyrin that he obtained from reduced hæmoglobin.

The feathers of *Turaco*, when placed in the path of a beam of light, show two well-marked absorption bands in the green portion of the spectrum. Possibly there is also another band, which is at best a very indistinct one, and as it may not be due to turacin we will disregard it, confining our attention to the obvious ones. These we will call α and β, the former having its position of maximum density at about 5830 Ångström units and the latter at about 5420 A.U. When the pigment is dissolved in, say, ·4 per cent. ammonia, the general character of the bands remains the same, but their positions alter. Each band shifts towards the blue end of the spectrum so that their new positions are $\alpha = 5625$ and $\beta = 5260$ A.U. It is not necessary that the turacin should be in the feathers however to give the former

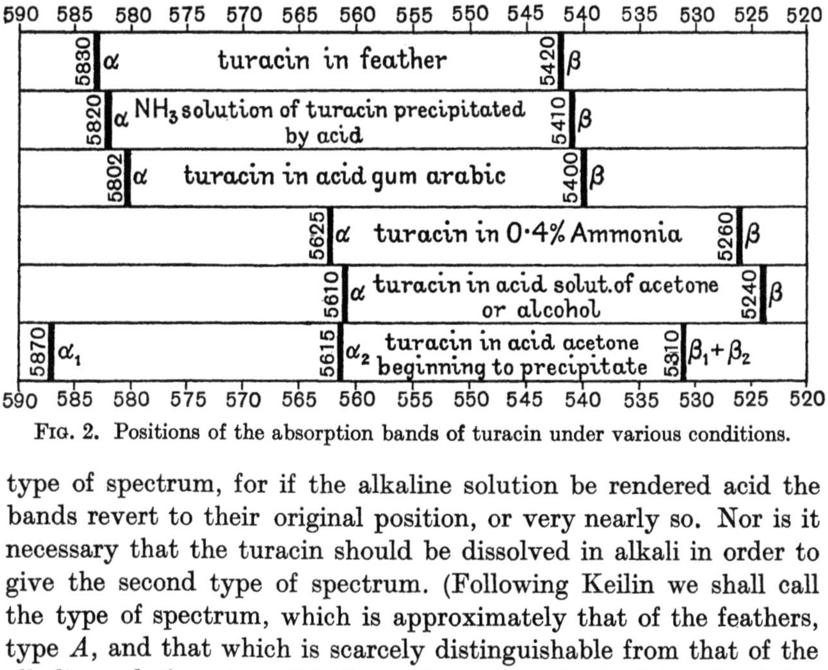

590	585	580	575	570	565	560	555	550	545	540	535	530	525	520

5830 α turacin in feather   5420 β

5820 α NH$_3$ solution of turacin precipitated by acid   5410 β

5802 α turacin in acid gum arabic   5400 β

5625 α turacin in 0·4% Ammonia   5260 β

5610 α turacin in acid solut. of acetone or alcohol   5240 β

5870 α_1 5615 α_2 turacin in acid acetone beginning to precipitate   5310 $\beta_1 + \beta_2$

590	585	580	575	570	565	560	555	550	545	540	535	530	525	520

FIG. 2. Positions of the absorption bands of turacin under various conditions.

type of spectrum, for if the alkaline solution be rendered acid the bands revert to their original position, or very nearly so. Nor is it necessary that the turacin should be dissolved in alkali in order to give the second type of spectrum. (Following Keilin we shall call the type of spectrum, which is approximately that of the feathers, type A, and that which is scarcely distinguishable from that of the alkaline solution, type B.) Type B may be obtained by dissolving turacin in acid alcohol, or in acid acetone. Indeed, according to Keilin, if the pigment be in true solution, whatever the solvent, type B is obtained, while type A appears only when the turacin is present in the form of a suspension. Thus the addition of acid to an alkaline solution of turacin precipitates the pigment at the same time that it alters the spectrum from type B to type A. There is a means, however, by which the precipitate may be retained in the form of a suspension, so fine that to the naked eye the appearance of a solution is simulated.

If some colloid material is present—gum arabic serves excellently for the purpose—in a solution of turacin in ·4 per cent. ammonia, the addition of acid does not now produce an obvious precipitate, the particles are "protected"—a phenomenon well known in colloid chemistry—by the colloid and give the appearance of being in solution whilst the type changes from B to A.

The points which I have tried to set forth are illustrated in the above figure. From above downwards are three conditions under which type A is found and then two under which type B appears. On looking at the figures the reader must remember that the charts are very far from representing photographs of the spectra, the lines shown are only a few Ångström units in width and represent as nearly as may be the position of maximum density of the bands. The bands themselves are broad, but it is not possible to say how broad, because that depends on the concentration of the solution, the intensity of the illumination, etc. With these points in mind let us consider what will occur if a solution of turacin is made slowly to precipitate.

To start with, before the precipitation commences only type B will be seen. As the precipitation proceeds a spectrum of type A will appear and will be superposed on type B. Now because the α-bands are relatively narrow and because the α-band of type A is widely separated from that of type B, the composite spectrum will show two α-bands which I shall call α_A and α_B. But in the composite spectrum β_A and β_B overlap, so that one band is seen in the β position, with its position of maximum density intermediate between that of β_A and β_B. We then have for a time a three-banded spectrum in which, as the precipitation proceeds, the A elements increase in distinctness at the expense of the B elements until, in the end, the A elements only are visible.

So much for turacin. To what extent is it possible to show a similar phenomenon in the case of other metalloporphyrins? The only one of these which has been studied is the iron compound. If the reader will look on page 9 he will find the graphical formula for hæmin. In that formula the chlorine may be replaced by OH yielding a base $C_{34}H_{32}O_4N_4Fe.OH$ which in the absence of oxygen may be reduced to $C_{34}H_{32}O_4N_4Fe$. The material so formed, like turacin, is soluble in alkali, but it is extremely insoluble in acid; the addition of acid therefore to the alkaline solution produces immediate precipitation. On the other hand, if acid be added to oxyhæmoglobin, a brown solution is obtained to which the name "acid hæmatin" has always been given. It would appear that the preparation is a solution in appearance only; it is really a suspension, the hæmatin being prevented, according to Keilin, from forming a gross precipitate by the protective action of the protein in which it is suspended. An exactly similar solution may be made from the base. If the hæmatin be dissolved in alkali, and to the solution a sufficient amount of gum arabic, gelatine or potassium silicate be added, then, on acidification, a suspension is formed which shows no tendency to precipitate and which gives a spectrum identical with that of the acid hæmatin made from oxyhæmoglobin.

With these phenomena in our minds we shall be in a stronger position to understand the nature of hæmoglobin and its related bodies. We must, however, undertake another preliminary enquiry, namely, one into the nature of hæmochromogen.

REFERENCES

(1) WILLSTÄTTER quoted Bayliss' *Principles of General Physiology*, 2nd ed. 561. 1918.

(2) VERNE, J. *Encyclop. Scient.* Doin Edit. 1926.

(3) MARCHELEWSKI, L. *Bull. Soc. Chim. Biol.* IV. 476. 1922.

(4) FISCHER, H. and his collaborators. Numerous studies published in the *Zeitsch. f. Physiol. Chemie* and *Liebig Annalen*, 1925–1926. A good résumé is to be found in the *Bulletin de la Société de Chimie Biologique*, VIII. 267. 1926.

(5) HILL, R. AND HOLDEN, H. F. *Biochem. Journ.* XX. 1326. 1926.

(6) LANKESTER, E. RAY. *Journ. Anat. and Physiol.* II. 114. 1867.

(7) FOX, H. MUNRO. *Proc. Roy. Soc. London*, B. XCIX. 199. 1925.

(8) LAIDLAW, P. P. *Journ. Physiol.* XXXI. 464. 1904.

(9) SCHULZ. *Arch. f. Anat. u. Physiol.* Suppl. 271. 1904.

(10) MILROY. *Journ. Physiol.* XXXVIII. 384. 1909.

(11) HILL, R. *Biochem. Journ.* XIX. 341. 1925.

(12) CHURCH. *Proc. Roy. Soc. London*, LI. 399. 1892; and *Phil. Trans.* B. CLXXXIII. 511. 1892.

(13) KEILIN, D. *Proc. Roy. Soc. London*, B. C. 129. 1926.

CHAPTER III

HÆMOCHROMOGEN

'HÆMOCHROMOGEN" and "reduced alkaline hæmatin" have been names hitherto attached on the one hand to a substance to which the formula $C_{34}H_{30}N_4O_4Fe$ has been given and on the other to a spectrum supposed to be the spectrum of that substance. Let us say a word or two firstly about the formula and secondly about the spectrum.

The formula is that of a protein-free substance: it is closely allied to hæmin ($C_{34}H_{30}N_4O_4FeCl$), and as there is no ambiguity about what hæmin is let us start with it. Hæmin is a chloride, it is of course obtained by acting on blood with glacial acetic acid and sodium chloride, which reaction, if properly carried out, produces the crystals known as Teichmann's crystals. These are crystals of hæmin and to them is given the formula $C_{34}H_{30}N_4O_4FeCl$. If the crystals are treated with caustic soda a base is liberated with the formula $C_{34}H_{30}N_4O_4FeOH$, and this base when reduced yields $C_{34}H_{30}N_4O_4Fe$—which has been our conception of reduced alkaline hæmatin. To turn now to the spectrum, one is always accustomed to tell students that the spectrum of hæmochromogen can be seen in extremely dilute solutions of the pigment. For this reason, among others, it is much sought after by those who specialise in the pursuit of blood stains on rags. The stain is extracted with caustic soda or potash, the coloured extract is reduced, and if the reduced fluid shows the "hæmochromogen" band the stain is assumed to have been blood.

The simple theory that hæmochromogen, yielding the characteristic spectrum, was the body $C_{34}H_{30}N_4O_4Fe$ obtained by the reduction of hæmatin $C_{34}H_{30}N_4O_4FeOH$, has been found by several observers, notably Bertin-Sans and Moitessier[1] and also Dilling[2], not to represent the whole truth.

They stated that during the reduction the presence of some nitrogenous body was necessary: what rôle this nitrogenous body played, whether it was a catalyst or a substance which entered in some more definite way into the reaction, was not stated by Bertin-Sans and Moitessier. Dilling was more explicit. He published his work in the form of a rather elaborate monograph, printed in English and in German with the same cover, and his spectroscopic constants are very carefully set out. He states definitely that hæmochromogen in his view is a chemical compound of hæmatin (a salt or ester with a nitrogenous substance). Yet the monograph was inaccessible, was apparently little read, and got buried. In spite of its publication the teaching three years ago was simply that when hæmatin ($C_{34}H_{30}N_4O_4FeOH$) was reduced, reduced alkaline hæmatin ($C_{34}H_{30}N_4O_4Fe$) was obtained, and that this body was identical with the substance hæmochromogen obtained by making blood alkaline and then reducing it, and therefore that the characteristic spectrum of hæmochromogen was a property of the material.

So the matter stood when it was taken up in 1924 by Anson and Mirsky[3]. Their line of approach was an enquiry as to whether the slight differences in the spectra of the hæmoglobins of various forms of life were reflected in the spectra of the hæmochromogens obtained by reducing these hæmoglobins in alkaline solution—Anson and Mirsky being under the impression that the hæmochromogens were protein-free substances.

It soon appeared that the spectrum with the conspicuous band, and the formula $C_{34}H_{30}N_4O_4Fe$, did not belong to the same substance. The formula was an attribute of one substance, the spectrum of another. Which shall we designate by the term "hæmochromogen"? Anson and Mirsky decided to keep the term "hæmochromogen" for the material with the conspicuous band, in which case it could no longer be applied to the substance with the formula $C_{34}H_{30}N_4O_4Fe$.

What then is the mistake which hitherto has vitiated our views and made us attach the formula of one substance to the spectrum of another? The mistake is that we have not recognised that hæmochromogen, prepared directly from hæmoglobin, like hæmoglobin itself, is a conjugated protein.

Suppose hæmochromogen be made in the way which has been indicated by rendering blood alkaline and then by reducing the alkaline fluid, it is clear that the protein is all present. The world supposed that it had been split off from the iron-containing portion of hæmoglobin, but the fact remains that any rigid separation of the globin from the pigment means the loss of the hæmochromogen spectrum.

On the other hand, if $C_{34}H_{30}N_4O_4Fe$ be made from the crystals of hæmin, the substance produced does not possess the spectrum of hæmochromogen. Add globin to it in sufficient quantity and the typical hæmochromogen spectrum appears.

It may seem strange that such a discrepancy between the facts and the interpretation put upon them could have passed unnoticed for so many years. There is one fact which possibly goes some way towards explaining the muddle and at the same time casts a flood of light on the whole subject. We have said above that $C_{34}H_{30}N_4O_4FeOH$ is the base obtained by the treatment of hæmin crystals with caustic soda or caustic potash. Ammonia was also frequently used for the liberation of the base for which purpose it is very good, but when the base is reduced in the presence of excess of ammonia that alkali, unlike KOH, has the further effect of uniting with the reduced hæmatin to form a corresponding hæmochromogen. Indeed, in the days of

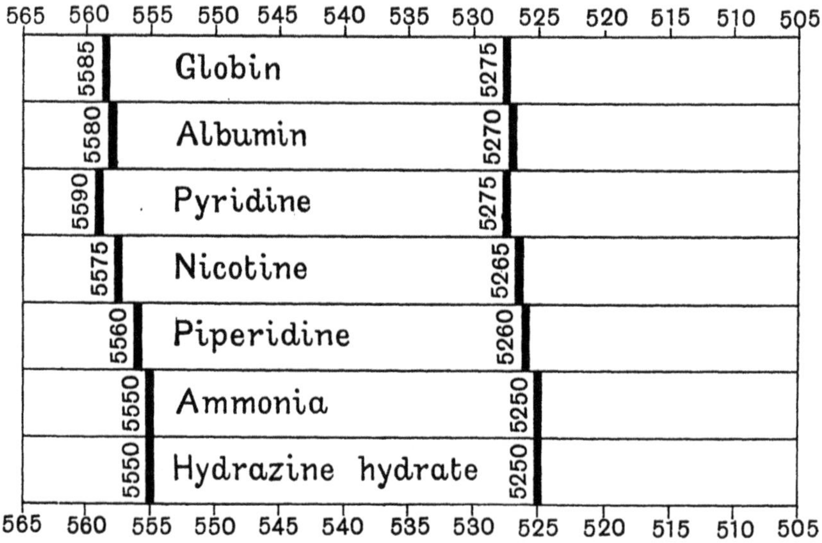

FIG. 3. Position of maximum density of bands in spectra of certain hæmochromogens.

more primitive spectrum analysis, the spectra of the ammonia body and of the protein body might have passed for the same. To-day it is clear that though not identical they are spectra of the same family. The bands are of the same general character in both spectra but their positions are somewhat different. Ammonia clearly has played the rôle both of the strong alkali and of the globin. It has liberated the base from the hæmin and, having liberated it, has made with the reduced hæmatin a conjugated nitrogenous body.

It is natural to suppose that if two bodies at the extreme ends of the scale, such as the simple body ammonia and the complicated globin molecule, can play the same part with regard to the base $C_{34}H_{30}N_4O_4Fe$, other molecules intermediate in complexity can do likewise. And this is so. Nicotine, pyridine, hydrazine hydrate, glycocol, and in fact many amines, some amino-acids and most of the proteins, will behave in the same way. The spectra of the hæmochromogens formed are all of the same character but differ in detail.

Here a word must be said about nomenclature. The following names were introduced by Anson and Mirsky starting from the view that hæmochromogen was a conjugated protein, obtained by making hæmoglobin alkaline and then adding a reducing agent. Anson and Mirsky having established the fact that hæmochromogen was an intermediate body between reduced hæmoglobin and $C_{34}H_{30}N_4O_4Fe$, not unnaturally applied the same line of reasoning to the compounds on the level of oxyhæmoglobin, in which case the apparently rich solution of pigment obtained by the addition of acid or alkali to oxyhæmoglobin would have ranged itself as a conjugated protein, which might have been prepared by the addition of protein to $C_{34}H_{30}N_4O_4FeOH$. While there is little doubt that such a view was in the minds of these authors and is certainly implied by them, it must be clearly stated that they do not claim to have carried out these transformations.

The following are Anson and Mirsky's schemes:

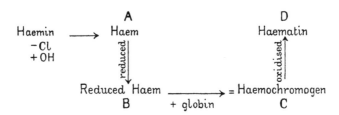

Anson and Mirsky did, however, stress one difference between "hæmatin" and "hæm," namely, the difference in solubility, and their observation was evident enough when demonstrated, particularly in acid solution. When acid is added to blood a dark brown solution is formed with the spectrum of hæmatin which is given in the text-books. When Teichmann's crystals (hæmin) are treated with NaOH and the solution rendered acid a precipitate gradually forms; it goes on forming until the whole of the pigment is precipitated. The natural inference would be that hæmatin in acid solution was very soluble whilst hæm in an acid medium was extremely insoluble.

Just at this point Keilin[4] made the interesting observation referred to in Chapter II that the apparent difference between the "hæm" and the "hæmatin" in acid was a question of environment. The reason why hæmatin produced by the addition of acid to blood does not come down is because the particles when formed are surrounded by a protective colloid which keeps them in suspension. If "acid hæm" be made as Anson and Mirsky made it but in a solution of about 0·2 per cent. gum arabic instead of an aqueous solution the "hæm" which is formed presents the general properties of "acid hæmatin," it remains in solution and gives the same spectrum as hæmatin. It must be concluded that "hæm" and "hæmatin" are the same substance. This discovery naturally raises the question of whether there is any great difference between reduced hæm and hæmochromogen, but here Keilin has entirely confirmed Anson and Mirsky, and of course it was the fact of hæmochromogen being a conjugated protein which constituted the essential point of Anson and Mirsky's work.

If the substance $C_{34}H_{30}N_4O_4FeOH$ which bears the names "hæm" and "hæmatin" be made in gum arabic so that the identity is evident and then reduced the reduced product is just what Anson and Mirsky described as reduced hæm so far as may be judged from its spectrum, and bears just the relation to hæmochromogen which Anson and Mirsky discovered. Keilin therefore calls in question the existence of a conjugated protein corresponding to Anson and Mirsky's "alkaline hæmatin," he believes that when alkali is added to blood the protein is broken off the iron porphyrin portion, for which he retains the word "hæmatin," and that therefore $C_{34}H_{30}N_4O_4Fe$ and protein are formed. Keilin believes further that when the mixture is reduced the protein and the iron porphyrin nucleus unite to form hæmochromogen. His scheme is as follows:

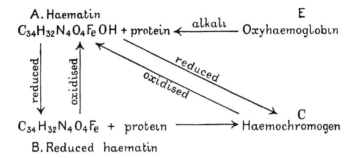

A. Haematin
$C_{34}H_{32}N_4O_4Fe\,OH$ + protein ← alkali — Oxyhaemoglobin   E

reduced | oxidised   reduced / oxidised

$C_{34}H_{32}N_4O_4Fe$ + protein ⟶ Haemochromogen   C

B. Reduced haematin

On the two schemes the bodies represented by the letters A, B, C, etc. are identical, whatever names are attached to them. D on Anson and Mirsky's scheme is, according to Keilin, non-existent in acid and alkaline solutions. In neutral solutions, however, there is admittedly a conjugated protein which corresponds to an oxidised form of hæmochromogen and which would occupy the position assigned to hæmatin by Anson and Mirsky. This body has a spectrum quite different from anything which is obtained from the oxidation of hæmochromogen in alkaline solution. The substance has been noticed by more than one observer. By v. Klaveren (5) it was called "kathæmoglobin," by Keilin (4), who has appreciated its real structure, it has been called "parahæmatin."

In what follows I shall adopt the nomenclature of Keilin and of Hill and Holden (6), retaining hæmatin for the base $C_{34}H_{30}N_4O_4FeOH$, reduced hæmatin for the base $C_{34}H_{30}N_4O_4Fe$, and hæmochromogen for the conjugated protein obtained by adding a nitrogenous substance to the latter. Having grasped the essential point, namely, that hæmochromogen is made by the addition of globin to the base $C_{34}H_{30}N_4O_4Fe$, it is desirable to look into the reaction more particularly. The fact is worth emphasis that the reaction is a balanced one. The equilibrium between a hæmochromogen and its constituents may be described in general terms as follows:

reduced hæmatin + nitrogenous compound ⇌ hæmochromogen.

The most obvious example is

reduced hæmatin + NH_3 ⇌ NH_3 hæmochromogen.

If this description is correct it must be possible by a suitable alteration in the relative concentrations of the reacting substances to make the equilibrium go in either direction. An increase in the concentration of hæmochromogen, on the addition of either reduced hæmatin or ammonia, may be demonstrated in the following way. The position of maximum density of the principal band in the spectrum of ammonia hæmochromogen is 35 Ångström units nearer the blue end than that of the corresponding band of globin hæmochromogen. If two vessels are placed in the beam of light of a Hartridge reversion spectroscope, one containing ammonia hæmochromogen and the other containing globin hæmochromogen, the band will appear to be in a position intermediate between those of the pure ammonia and the pure globin compounds. The exact position depends upon the relative concentration of the two compounds. Thus if the concentration of the globin compound be increased the band shifts towards the red, if the concentration of the ammonia compound be increased the band shifts towards the blue. Start then with the combined band in a certain definite position and add reduced hæmatin to the solution which contains the ammonia hæmochromogen. The band at once shifts towards the violet showing that the concentration of ammonia hæmochromogen in the fluid has increased. In a solution of hæmochromogen what proportion does the concentration of hæmochromogen bear to those of the reduced hæmatin and the globin which are present? The precise answer is not known. The combination is almost complete, the concentrations of hæmatin and globin being very small relatively to the concentration of hæmochromogen. When the whole range of hæmochromogens is reviewed the fact emerges that globin hæmochromogen is an exception in this respect. Contrast it with ammonia hæmochromogen. To obtain that substance it is necessary to add an overwhelming amount of ammonia to the reduced hæmatin. So far, indeed, out of all the nitrogenous compounds which have been found to unite with reduced hæmatin two only have affinities for it at all approaching that of globin. The two are pyridine and nicotine. Globin, then, among the nitrogenous compounds which could unite with hæmatin, has a very special place, if only because it is one of the few substances which have a great affinity for hæmatin.

Hæmatin is a very insoluble substance, and a second respect in which globin presents an especial interest is that it forms a vehicle for the conversion of the insoluble hæmatin into a soluble compound.

Let us now pass to the consideration of the nature of hæmoglobin in the light of what we know of hæmochromogen. What is the relation of the one to the other? Several workers have claimed the distinction of having prepared hæmoglobin; they may have done so but until recently there has been great difficulty in repeating these preparations. Indeed they cannot claim to have stood the test of repetition. Quite lately, however, claims have been put forward both by Anson and Mirsky and by Hill and Holden[6] to have prepared hæmoglobin and by completely different methods. The evidence is entirely spectroscopic. It is not claimed by Anson and Mirsky that the crystalline oxyhæmoglobin was obtained, nor is that claim made by Hill and Holden. What I ask of both is that they should produce the material (and preferably in the crystalline form) in sufficient quantity for me to determine the dissociation curve! The point on which Hill and Holden lay stress is that the globin used must be of the particular type known as "undenatured"—I must admit that to me this word was once a little frightening. The globin is prepared from oxyhæmoglobin and the precautions necessary to prevent its denaturation are fully set out in Hill and Holden's paper. When added to hæmatin (made by dissolving hæmin in sodium carbonate) methæmoglobin results. The remaining processes are familiar: methæmoglobin treated with a reducing agent gives reduced hæmoglobin which when oxidised yields oxyhæmoglobin. Not only have Hill and Holden made ordinary oxyhæmoglobin in this way but, using the same undenatured protein, they have attached it to the analogues of hæmatin made not from protoporphyrin but from hæmato- and mesoporphyrins, and so obtained the hæmoglobins, the spectra of which were described in the last chapter. No small performance I think.

REFERENCES

(1) BERTIN-SANS AND MOITESSIER. *C. R. Ac. Sci. Paris,* CXVI. 591. 1893.

(2) DILLING. *Atlas of Hœmochromogens.* Stuttgart, 1910. *Atlas der Krystallformen u. Absorptionbänder der Hämochromogene.*

(3) ANSON, BARCROFT, MIRSKY AND OINUMA. *Proc. Roy. Soc.* B. XCVII. 61. 1925. ANSON AND MIRSKY. *Journ. Physiol.* LX. 50. 1925.

(4) KEILIN. *Proc. Roy. Soc.* B. C. 129. 1926.

(5) v. KLAVEREN. *Zeit. Physiol. Chem.* XXXIII. 293. 1901.

(6) HILL AND HOLDEN. *Biochem. Journ.* XX. 1326. 1926.

CHAPTER IV

CYTOCHROME

I⊤ is a fit subject for remark, if not for surprise, how few organic substances figure prominently in both the animal and vegetable kingdoms. One of the few is cytochrome, a substance which has only recently been placed in its present important setting by the researches of Keilin [1]. Perhaps it is too much even to call it a substance, for it may occur, as the seedsmen's catalogues say, "in variety," but if we regard cytochrome merely as the name for a spectrum, that spectrum is sufficiently widespread in its occurrence to justify the name being placed at the head of the fourth chapter of this book.

Let us turn to the spectrum and having gained familiarity with it let us then discuss its significance.

If the wing muscles of a bee be laid out on a glass slide in a thin layer and exposed to air and looked at with a microspectroscope, no particular spectrum will be seen. But if the muscles be covered over with a slide, or otherwise protected from the oxygen of the air, a band shortly appears; in time this band becomes more intense, and other bands, ultimately three of them, come into view till at last a spectrum is seen which undergoes no further change. This spectrum consists of four bands of different degrees of intensity, that seen first being the most intense. It is the spectrum of cytochrome.

Cytochrome is readily oxidised in the living cells, and in the oxidised form it has but a poor spectrum. Therefore in the bee's muscle exposed to air, the cytochrome being present in the oxidised form, the absorption bands are hardly perceptible when such a preparation is viewed through the microspectroscope. When, however, a coverslip is placed on the muscle, especially if the latter be in fluid, the muscular material reduces the cytochrome and, as the concentration of reduced cytochrome increases, the bands appear, the most intense naturally being the first to make its appearance.

That the number of bands really depends upon the quantity of cytochrome in the layer of muscle traversed by the light on its way through the instrument, may be demonstrated in a very simple way.

When the experiment which has already been described has been performed (the cover glass being of sufficient strength), and all four bands are clearly seen, press on the cover glass so as gradually to decrease the thickness of the layer of muscle. In proportion as the layer becomes thinner the bands will disappear, one by one, in the reverse order to that in which they appeared. At last only the most prominent band in the cytochrome spectrum remains visible.

The four bands of the cytochrome from bee's muscle have their positions of maximum density placed as follows:

band $a = 6046$ A.U., $b = 5665$ A.U., $c = 5502$ A.U., $d = 5210$ A.U.

The facts described above illustrate the ease with which mistakes may be made in the quest of such spectra. A spectrum in some new object might be seen with one, two, three or four bands. Such might be described as different spectra and attributed to the presence of different materials but these apparently diverse spectra would be caused merely by different dilutions of a single substance having a spectrum with four bands of different densities. It may be said

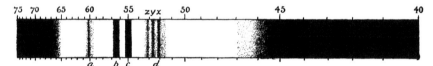

Fig. 4. Spectrum of absorption of cytochrome in the thoracic muscles of the bee.

at once that in no material in which the c-band has been seen have the other three bands failed to appear when the material has been concentrated, or rather the layer of material thickened to the adequate extent; and as the c-band of cytochrome is one of great intensity it soon came to be recognised by Keilin as a sort of label for the whole spectrum, a fact which greatly facilitated his researches into the widespread distribution of this material.

So far we have considered bee's muscle because in the bee we have a creature which is uncomplicated by the presence of hæmoglobin. The same is true of many other forms of animal life.

The following list, showing the wide distribution of cytochrome, is given by Keilin:

Turbellaria.	*Dendrocela lactea.*
Oligochætes.	*Allolobophora chlorotica, Helodrilus caliginosus.*
Nematodes.	*Ascaris megalocephala, Ascaris suis.*
Molluscs.	*Limnea peregra, L. stagnalis, Helix nemoralis, H. aspersa.*
Crustacea.	*Oniscus sp., Asellus aquaticus, Cancer pagurus.*
Myriapods.	*Lithobius forficatus.*

ARACHNIDS.   *Epeira diademata.*

INSECTS.   About forty species have been examined, all of which contain cytochrome, among which are the house-fly, the lesser house-fly, the blow-fly, the tsetse-fly, *Gastrophilus intestinalis, Eristalis tenax, Anopheles maculipennis, Culex pipiens,* the hornet, wasp, bumble-bee, honey-bee, silkworm moth, wax moth, etc.

VERTEBRATES.   Cytochrome was found in the tissues of fish, frog, pigeon, guinea-pig, rabbit and sheep.

Perhaps the most exciting excursion of Keilin's work is that which took him into the vegetable kingdom. For the cytochrome spectrum may be found in a great number of plants ranging from the lowest to the highest forms. It may be seen in yeast, equally it may be seen in the onion and in certain aerobic bacteria. Thus it is to be found in the animal kingdom right down through every phylum to the worms, and in the vegetable kingdom from the bacterium right up to the flowering plant—surely a sufficiently universal distribution.

Fig. 5 gives the position of the cytochrome bands in a number of typical forms.

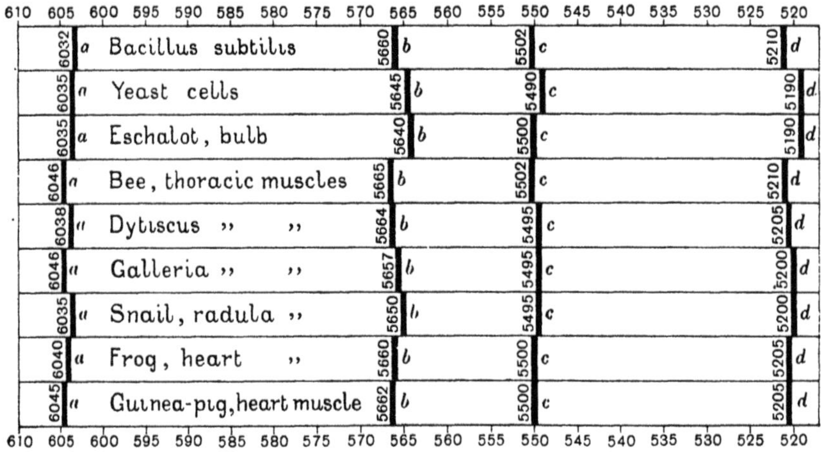

Source	Band *a*	Band *b*	Band *c*	Band *d*
Bacillus subtilis	6032	5660	5502	5210
Yeast cells	6035	5645	5490	5190
Eschalot, bulb	6035	5640	5500	5190
Bee, thoracic muscles	6046	5665	5502	5210
Dytiscus ,, ,,	6038	5664	5495	5205
Galleria ,, ,,	6046	5657	5495	5200
Snail, radula ,,	6035	5650	5495	5200
Frog, heart ,,	6040	5660	5500	5205
Guinea-pig, heart muscle	6045	5662	5500	5205

FIG. 5. Spectra of cytochrome from various sources in the animal and vegetable kingdoms.

An inspection of Fig. 5 will show why I had some misgivings about saying that cytochrome was identical in all forms of life. A detailed analysis shows that going from form to form the whole spectrum is now a few Ångström units to the right, now a few to the left, the largest divergence being in band *b*, that between eschalot and bee, and amounting to 25 A.U.

Baker's yeast represents by far the best material for study of oxidation and reduction of cytochrome:

If a shallow tube (30 mm. high) is half-filled with a suspension of baker's yeast (20 per cent.) in water and the suspension is examined with a Zeiss microspectroscope, the four absorption bands may be clearly seen; but when air is rapidly bubbled through the suspension the cytochrome becomes oxidised and the bands disappear. If the current of air is stopped the pigment becomes reduced and the four bands rapidly reappear. A similar result can be obtained by shaking a 5 c.c. yeast emulsion in a test-tube and examining it with the microspectroscope. When, instead of air, a current of N_2 is passed through the yeast emulsion or when the latter is shaken with N_2, the cytochrome remains in reduced state showing all the time its four characteristic absorption bands.

Cytochrome cannot be regarded as an alternative to hæmoglobin, for in muscles the two pigments are found together. Take for instance the muscle of a perfused guinea-pig; it was here really that Keilin started his researches. If this muscle be treated in the way which has already been described, the muscle being looked at in air through the microspectroscope, the spectrum of O_2-hæmoglobin is seen. It is true that the position of the bands is not precisely the same as in the hæmoglobin of guinea-pig's blood: the finer points of the placing of hæmoglobin bands must be left to the future for discussion. Here it need only be said that the bands seen in guinea-pig's muscle are precisely similar to the bands presented by the hæmoglobin of the larva of *Gastrophilus*—a parasite which is found in the stomach of the horse. But to continue the experiment: shortly after the cover glass is put on, the bands change abruptly. The two bands of O_2-hæmoglobin give place to the four-banded spectrum of cytochrome. The uninitiated might easily be excused for the supposition that a single pigment was present which gave a two-banded spectrum when oxidised and a four-banded spectrum when reduced. Or in less concentration, a two-banded spectrum when oxidised and a one-, two- or three-banded spectrum when reduced. It would be futile here to hark back to the polemic[2] as between MacMunn or Hoppe-Seyler, or to investigate the cloud of obscurity which has enveloped the pigments in mammalian muscle since their time. The simple fact, however, is that all the spectral phenomena of guinea-pig's muscle may be imitated, if a suitable mixture be made of sheep's blood hæmoglobin and yeast emulsion. When this mixture is shaken with air and rapidly examined with the microspectroscope it shows only the two bands of oxyhæmoglobin, while the cytochrome of the yeast, being oxidised, does not show the absorption bands. Keeping the mixture under observation, both pigments become rapidly reduced, the bands of oxyhæmoglobin disappear, being replaced by faint bands of reduced hæmoglobin, while the bands of the reduced cytochrome rapidly appear.

Here we are faced with a phenomenon which will crop up later, with regard for instance to hæmochromogen and hæmoglobin; and just as we use the word "hæmoglobin" to cover the whole range of substances which possess spectra approximately, but not precisely identical, so we will retain the word "cytochrome" to cover a similar range of substances which have approximately the spectrum shown in Fig. 4. The sorts of differences which occur are shown in Fig. 5.

It may not have escaped the reader, especially if he be an organic chemist, that such information as I have given about cytochrome has all been gleaned by the inspection of living cells, and that neither the name cytochrome nor the four-banded spectrum represents a substance which has been isolated. I will not enter into the question of how far a material which has not been isolated can be regarded as satisfactory. I will at once concede to the organic chemist of the purist school that such a material is less satisfactory than if it had been isolated, but I must claim for those who are prepared to study "life as a whole" that a man places an undue limitation on his intellect if he is not prepared to look at living things as they are, but will merely study the artifacts about which he can obtain more precise information. Suffice it to say that the component cytochrome has not been isolated, but although this is so the attempt has furnished important information which goes some way to show where cytochrome stands in relation especially to hæmoglobin.

The spectrum of cytochrome has been described as having four bands, but one of these bands, d, when carefully examined with a Zeiss microspectroscope is found to be in reality composed of three bands which are more or less merged. The cytochrome spectrum has therefore six bands which are related to one another in an interesting way. We will call them, not a, b, c and d, but a, b, c, z, y and x. These six bands may be seen in Fig. 4 in which the tripartite nature of the band d is well shown. One remarkable property about the six bands is that they appear to be related to one another in pairs. To start with the consideration of a, b and c. These three bands are not always of the same relative intensity. As has been said, c is usually much the most conspicuous and a the least so. In the wing muscles of the bumble-bee [3], however, a is of unusual relative intensity; in the muscles which operate the radula of the edible snail b is unusually prominent as compared with a and c. In baker's yeast also band b is as conspicuous as band c. Now to pass to bands x, y and z. Where band c is conspicuous relatively to a and b, band x is conspicuous relatively to z and y, similarly z pairs off with a and y with b, so that in the bumble-bee z is relatively intense, whilst in the snail's tongue-muscle and in baker's yeast, y is more prominent than is ordinarily the case.

This pairing of the bands suggests that the spectrum of cytochrome is not that of a single substance but of a mixture of three substances, of which bands a and z represent the spectrum of one, b and y of the second, and c and x of the third. Each substance would then have a two-banded spectrum (Fig. 6). Let us see what further evidence there may be for this tripartite structure of cytochrome. Is it possible to

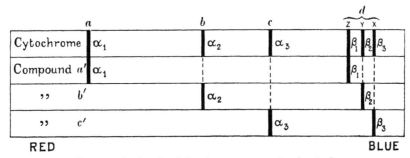

Fig. 6. Showing the bands of the three components of cytochrome.

abolish one pair of bands without abolishing the whole? This may be done. As has been said oxidation of cytochrome under ordinary circumstances abolishes all the bands, but if a suspension of baker's yeast be treated with urethane or alcohol before oxidation the bands disappear *seriatim* when the suspension is oxidised; of the bands a, b and c, c disappears first (with it x), then a (with z), so that b, of these three, remains alone with the corresponding part of d.

Again, if yeast be dried and the dried mass be extracted with water a yellowish opalescent liquid results. This liquid shows only two bands, one of which corresponds to band c, and the other to a portion of the band d of cytochrome. It may be inferred therefore that the aqueous extract of the desiccated yeast contains one and one only of the three constituents of cytochrome.

Now a fresh light flashes on the constitution of cytochrome—surely this two-banded spectrum of the aqueous extract is a very old friend—

it is none other than hæmochromogen; but in what company to
meet it! Sherlock Holmes himself could not make a more dramatic
appearance than that of a blood pigment in a mixed company of
yeast cells, bacteria and onions.

If then we can derive a hæmochromogen from cytochrome is it
possible to derive a cytochrome spectrum from hæmochromogen?
Seemingly that can be accomplished. At all events a family of
characteristic spectra can be obtained by treating various hæmochromogens with potassium ferricyanide. These spectra differ no
more from cytochrome than the cytochrome spectra from various
sources differ from one another—as is shown in Fig. 7. The upper-
most two spectra are those of the cytochromes of yeast and of
guinea-pig's muscle; the three lower ones are obtained by the alternate
treatment, with potassium ferricyanide and a reducer, of nicotine-
hæmochromogen, pyridine-hæmochromogen and globin-hæmochromogen respectively.

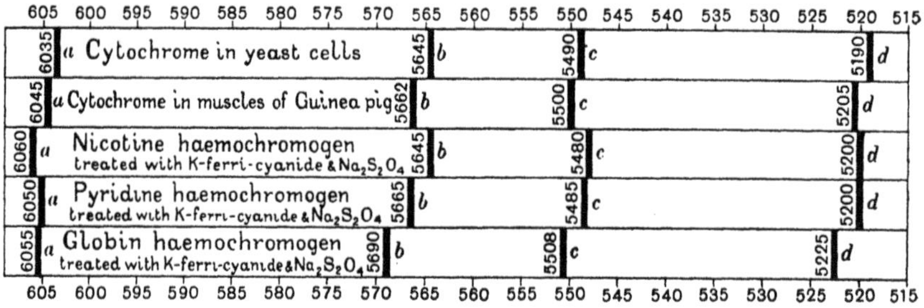

FIG. 7.

If, as the foregoing observations seem to suggest, hæmochromogen
is closely connected with cytochrome the question naturally arises:
Is it possible to find either hæmochromogen or hæmatin in cells
which subsequently contain cytochrome, but which never contain
hæmoglobin? The answer is that hæmatin may be so found, both in
cells which will one day contain cytochrome and in cells which
actually do contain cytochrome. This is true not only of the animal
but of the vegetable kingdom. The whole history may be seen in the
blow-fly:

If one examines spectroscopically the larva of such a fly one sees that the adipose
tissue holds a great quantity of hæmatin and a little ordinary hæmochromogen whilst
the larval muscles in addition to free hæmatin contain cytochrome. During the
metamorphosis the quantity of free hæmatin in the adipose tissues gradually diminishes,

whilst the concentration of cytochrome, especially in the muscles, increases. The thoracic muscles of the pupa, and still more of the imago ready to hatch, contain a great proportion of cytochrome in addition to a little hæmatin. In the same way the free hæmatin of the endosperm of grass seed or of the reserve tissues of other plants can store material for the formation of the hæmochromogen and of the cytochrome appearing in the cells which are carrying on an active metabolism (4).

The fact is that hæmatin is a substance of very wide distribution. The reason why its presence has been unsuspected is that it is not at all easily seen, not being a body with sharp spectral bands. Our new knowledge of hæmochromogen, however, teaches us how to turn the inconspicuous hæmatin into the conspicuous hæmochromogen—that is done by the addition of pyridine in the presence of a reducer. Indeed hæmatin may be demonstrated in the presence of cytochrome by converting the hæmatin into CO-hæmatin and then adding pyridine. Hæmatin is present in quite ordinary articles (3), (4) of vegetable diet—in wheaten flour and oaten meal for instance. It seems remarkable enough that mankind, in what he has been pleased to call the staff of life, has for countless centuries been eating, all unknowingly, the outstanding constituent of his blood.

Something remains to be said about the nature of the transformation from hæmochromogen to cytochrome. It takes place in the plant; it can be made to take place in the test-tube by the alternate reduction and oxidation (with ferricyanide) of the hæmochromogen and it is not dependent upon the protein since the spectra of the analogous nicotine and pyridine cytochromes can be made from the hæmochromogens in a similar way. The nature of the change from the hæmochromogen which contains natural hæmatin, to the cytochrome analogue, or possibly the three cytochrome analogues, is still obscure.

To commence with, there is but one natural hæmatin, and there appear to be three hæmochromogens in cytochrome. The easiest assumption is that one hæmatin is attached to three different nitrogenous moieties; this explanation is negatived by the fact that cytochrome may be obtained in which the nitrogenous moiety is in every case pyridine or in every case nicotine. It must be then that the hæmatin itself is altered. In Chapter II it was shown that the formation of almost any number of porphyrins was possible in theory. If therefore the porphyrin in hæmatin could be altered at all by successive oxidations and reductions, it might as easily be altered into three other porphyrins as one.

There is still the possibility, however, that one cytochrome consists of not more than two hæmochromogens: we have seen how these two spectra can be made from turacin or hæmatin according as it is in a state of colloid suspension or of true solution. A mixture of these two might easily give a three-banded spectrum, involving, say, the lines b, c and so much of d as was involved in y and x. This would leave only a and z to be accounted for by a second body. But we are still in the region of speculation where there is as yet no certain knowledge.

Here we must leave the constitution of cytochrome until further information is forthcoming, and turn to its function—a field no less exciting than that of its constitution or occurrence.

What cytochrome effects in the cell, appears to be bound up with the fact that the pigment itself is oxidisable when the cells containing it are exposed to air and reducible by reducing agents of the cells. To understand its function we must first grasp certain facts concerning the conditions under which the cytochrome acquires and parts with its oxygen. Of these the first is the influence of potassium cyanide upon the oxidation of the pigment. If bee's muscle or yeast be examined whilst precautions are taken to keep the air away from the material, as by putting a coverslip over it, the cytochrome will be reduced by the activity of the material itself. If now it be treated in the reduced condition with a very dilute ($N/10,000$) solution of potassium cyanide the spectrum of the reduced pigment becomes fixed, so that subsequent exposure to air does not wipe out the bands and therefore may be presumed not to oxidise the cytochrome. The action of potassium cyanide leads to one interesting phenomenon, namely, by invoking its aid the bands of oxyhæmoglobin and cytochrome may be obtained in the same solution. Under ordinary circumstances they cannot exist together because the oxyhæmoglobin band can only persist in the presence of a certain partial pressure of free oxygen, which if present oxidises the cytochrome. If, however, a mixture of cytochrome and hæmoglobin, both in the reduced condition, be treated with potassium cyanide and then shaken with air, the oxygen introduced will oxidise only the hæmoglobin, thus giving the oxyhæmoglobin bands without abolishing those of the cytochrome.

The reader should grasp the importance of the above observation. Potassium cyanide is of all reagents one of the most lethal. The text-book statement is that the cyanide prevents oxidation in the tissues. The fact is that in animals poisoned with cyanide the blood goes through the capillaries and enters the veins unreduced. Why? The possibility now presents itself that cytochrome provides a link in the chain of events which connects the loss of oxygen from the hæmoglobin with the actual building up of that gas into the tissue, and that if this link be broken by the potassium cyanide the oxidation process in the cell becomes much impaired. Such a conception would present cytochrome as a substance which was always taking up oxygen in the presence of oxidase and imparting it, not as free oxygen, but by some system of double decomposition, to the oxidisable materials in immediate contact with it.

It may seem to the reader that the claim of cytochrome to pose as a link in the oxidation process of the cell rests on too circumscribed a foundation, when it is based upon the relation of but one substance, potassium cyanide, to the pigment. Such diffidence is not out of place, and the investigations prompted by it have led to the discovery of some other interesting properties of cytochrome. Let us turn therefore to the consideration of a wholly different class of substances, which, however, resemble potassium cyanide in one respect, namely, that they reduce oxidation processes proper to vitality to the point of ultimate extinction. Such substances are general anæsthetics such as alcohol, chloroform, aldehydes, compound ureas, etc. It is remarkable that these, too, abolish the power of cytochrome to be alternately oxidised and reduced, and even more remarkable that they effect this immobilisation of the cytochrome in quite a different way from that in which potassium cyanide achieves the same end. The narcotics mentioned do not prevent the oxidation of the reduced cytochrome, on the other hand they prevent the reduction of the oxidised pigment, breaking the link as it were at the other end. Such an hypothesis is one which endows cytochrome with catalytic properties, and which leads one up to the question: Is cytochrome an important catalyst or only one of many which may be in the cell? Three sets of facts are worth noting with regard to the importance of cytochrome as a catalyst: (1) its distribution as related to the activity of the tissues in which it is found, (2) its claim to be a peroxidase, and (3) its position as a substance which contains iron. Let us discuss these three points.

1. *The distribution and behaviour of cytochrome in relation to the activity of the tissues in which it is found.* From numerous illustrations cited by Keilin the following may be quoted in support of his thesis that a general correspondence exists between the activity of a tissue

and the concentration of the cytochrome which is contained in its substance:

(1) Bacteria: aerobic bacteria, such as *Bacillus subtilis*, contain cytochrome or free hæmatin, while the anaerobic bacteria, *B. sporogenes*, are completely devoid of these pigments.

(2) Yeast. Baker's yeast has a much higher concentration of cytochrome than brewer's yeast. It was proved by Meyerhoff that in presence of glucose, baker's yeast uses ten times more oxygen than brewer's yeast.

(3) In snails, the greatest amount of cytochrome is found in the active muscles of radula.

(4) In crabs, the muscles of the body and of the appendages, which contract slowly, contain a small concentration of this pigment which is present in much higher concentration in the active and rhythmically contracting muscles of the heart.

(5) In frogs, the highest concentration of this pigment is found in the muscles of the heart.

(6) In birds which fly, the pectoral muscles and the muscles of the heart contain the greatest amount of this pigment.

(7) In rabbits, the order of concentration is: heart muscles, muscles connected with mastication, diaphragm, muscles of the legs, etc.

(8) The most interesting examples are, however, found among insects. The high concentration of cytochrome in their wing muscles is undoubtedly connected with the peculiar activity of these muscles, which are capable of producing up to 300 complete contractions per second. On the other hand, the thoracic muscles of wingless insects show only a very low concentration of this pigment. The best example is, however, shown by the winter moth (*Cheimatobia brumata*):

The male of this moth which is provided with well developed wings and flies well shows the presence of cytochrome clearly, while the female with reduced non-functional wings scarcely shows the pigment in the muscles.

Another case is that of the cockroach:

In cockroaches (*Stylopyga orientalis*) which do not fly, but are good runners, cytochrome is found specially in the muscles of the legs.

The last case has to do with the development of the fly:

Taking as an example the common blow-fly, we find that cytochrome is already present in the eggs and in the muscles of the larva. The concentration of the pigment in these muscles is found to be approximately ten to fifteen times lower than that in the thoracic muscles of the adult fly. During the metamorphosis the concentration of cytochrome in the freshly formed thoracic muscles of the pupa increases with its development. The adult insect, however, does not contain the maximum amount of pigment immediately on hatching. This is reached during adult life.

2. *The claim of cytochrome to be a peroxidase* is stated by Keilin as follows:

Cytochrome and its derivatives have the properties of a thermostable peroxidase. All the tissues when cytochrome is present and can be seen spectroscopically, give a good reaction with benzidine, and with guaiacum and hydrogen peroxide. The tissues of invertebrates where the pigment is very meagre give a very weak reaction or none at all. In a single individual, *Dytiscus* for example, the brown muscles, which are rich in cytochrome, give a strong positive peroxidase reaction, while the white muscles, which are very poor in cytochrome, give hardly any reaction.

3. No discussion of the significance of cytochrome can close without some reference to a problem which has fascinated biologists now for a quarter of a century, namely, the relation of the group of pigments in the animal kingdom, which finds its highest development in hæmoglobin, to that without which only the humblest forms of vegetable life exist, namely, chlorophyll. The fact of the pyrrol groupings existing in each has prompted the use of the word "Suggestive" with the largest possible capital S: hitherto, however, the suggestions have failed to yield the fruit of any biological relation between the two sets of pigments. Verne[5] has gone so far as to suppose that the hæmatin pigments of animal life are derived from the chlorophyll contained in the ingredients of the vegetable food. Now the facts must be orientated afresh: in more primitive forms of life than those in which either hæmoglobin or chlorophyll exist, there may be found the tetrapyrrol grouping in hæmatin and cytochrome. Yeast and bacteria for instance fed on media entirely free from chlorophyll exhibit the spectral bands of cytochrome and hæmatin. If chemical relationship and phylogeny have any thing to do with one another it is more probable that chlorophyll has been derived by the living organism from hæmatin than hæmatin from chlorophyll.

Is this "Suggestive"? The yellow portions of the leaf of *Euonymus* contain cytochrome, the green ones chlorophyll.

REFERENCES

(1) KEILIN. *Proc. Roy. Soc.* B. xcviii. 312. 1925.
(2) MacMUNN. *Phil. Trans. Roy. Soc.* clxxvii. 267. 1886.
(3) KEILIN. *Proc. Roy. Soc.* B. c. 129. 1926.
(4) KEILIN. *C. R. de la Soc. de Biol. Paris.* Réunion plénière, xcvii. 39. 1927.
(5) VERNE. "Les Pigments dans l'organisme animal." *Encyclop. Scient.* Doin, 1926.

CHAPTER V

THE SPECIFICITY OF HÆMOGLOBIN

In many text-books of physiology there will be seen a picture of crystals of the hæmoglobins of several animals. The moral of the picture is that these crystals differ in form. Yet within recent years very little attention has been paid to their differences, possibly because they were in no way linked up with the properties of the hæmoglobins as carriers of oxygen.

In 1909 the Carnegie Institute published a monumental report on the subject by Prof. Reichert, who held the chair of Physiology in Philadelphia, and his colleague, the professor of mineralogy in the same University, Dr A. S. Brown(1). The scope of the work may be judged from the fact that 600 different photographs of the crystals of hæmoglobin from different animals are published in the hundred plates at the end of the book, whilst in 338 quarto pages of letterpress the properties of these crystals are tabulated and discussed. Starting with the fishes, these authors go right up the vertebrate scale and end with an investigation of the blood of the primates. And yet there is much unsaid. There are many well-known forms of life, the hæmoglobin of which is not discussed. I need go no further than the frog. Why? Well, of course I can only speculate, but I suppose that they could not make the hæmoglobin from frog's blood crystallise. And here I would like to put in a plea for the publication of negative results. At the present time, when the claims on the space in journals are very great, it is natural to pass over experiments which have led to no positive result. Moreover a man of modest disposition feels that he is making rather a "fuss about nothing" in publishing his negative experiences, but all that is no comfort to his successor who, after much toil and labour, arrives at precisely the same point, only to be told that A, B or C had travelled the same road before him and with the same result. In the present case it would be very interesting to know what forms of life had yielded hæmoglobin which Reichert and Brown had found impossible to crystallise. The bare allusion to these facts brings out two properties, in addition to crystalline form, in which the different animals' hæmoglobins differ, namely, solubility and ease of crystallisation. Solubility will be dealt

with later in this chapter when the work of Landsteiner and Heidel-
berger(2) is discussed. With regard to ease of crystallisation we
may say at once that the hæmoglobin of different animals differs
greatly in this respect. Ordinary laboratory practice makes one
familiar with the difference between, say, the blood of the horse and
that of the ox. Hæmoglobin crystals can be obtained from the former
with ease, in fact it is only necessary to centrifuge horse blood in
a Sharpless separator, as used in Prof. L. J. Henderson's laboratory by
Ferry(3), to obtain them in profusion. On the other hand, quite
special methods are required to obtain crystals of ox hæmoglobin.
Or again, among the rodents, rabbit's blood crystallises with difficulty,
that of the guinea-pig with ease. And even among the rats, according
to Reichert and Brown, the oxyhæmoglobins of the Norway rat and
of the white rat are relatively insoluble, while those of the black and
Alexandrine rats are much more soluble.

The impression which one gets from this mass of information is:

(1) That no two hæmoglobins are quite the same.

(2) That even in the same animal there is more than one form of
hæmoglobin. Of these different hæmoglobins in one animal one type
is more easily crystallised than another; therefore, as crystallisation
progresses, two or three crops of crystals may appear. These are called
the α-, β- and γ-hæmoglobins. To quote Reichert and Brown:

For instance, in the baboons three distinct crops of crystal oxyhæmoglobin developed: (1) tabular and lath-shaped orthorhombic crystals, (2) short prismatic or
tabular monoclinic crystals, and (3) tabular orthorhombic crystals. It is possible
that (1) and (3) may be the same substance, but very unlikely; (2) is evidently a
different substance. In the same genus two forms of methæmoglobin were observed,
one orthorhombic and one monoclinic, corresponding to the α- and β-hæmoglobins....
Among the rodents two forms of hæmoglobin were observed in a number of species....
Thus, in the blood of the domestic rabbit an orthorhombic and a monoclinic form of
oxyhæmoglobin are found that are evidently different.

The crystals of hæmoglobin are also dimorphous in the horse, the
marmot and many other animals.

Crystals of the species of any genus belong to the same crystallographic system
and generally to the same crystallographic group; and they have approximately the
same axial ratios, or their ratios are in simple relation to each other. In other words,
the hæmoglobin crystals of any genus are isomorphous. In some cases the isomorphism
may be extended to include several genera, but this is not usually the case, unless,
as in the case of the dogs and foxes for example, the genera are very closely related....

Where several kinds of hæmoglobin are to be looked for in one
species of a genus, they are to be looked for in other species of the

same genus, and where conditions are favourable they can presumably all be developed in each species.

Some interesting facts which may bear upon the relations of different species and genera to one another are recorded. Among the primates for instance, the α-oxyhæmoglobin of the baboon and of man are strikingly alike; the β-oxyhæmoglobin of the baboon has no counterpart in man but the γ-oxyhæmoglobin in the two are similar.

Among the rats:

It has been generally stated in the zoologies that the white rat is an albino of the black rat. From our examination of the crystals it is evident that the white rat is closely related to the brown or Norway rat, but it cannot be closely related to the black or Alexandrine rat.

Again, by some zoologists the bats have been placed among the primates and the relationship of the groups has been claimed by a number of zoologists. The crystals of oxyhæmoglobin from the brown bat do show a considerable resemblance to the crystals of oxyhæmoglobin of the genus *Papio*, but on the other hand the fruit-bat examined showed quite a different type of crystal.

Specific differences in the solubilities of the hæmoglobins of different animals have been the subject of a fascinating research by Landsteiner and Heidelberger [2]. These differences are no less striking than the differences of crystalline form, and are no doubt related to the ease with which hæmoglobin crystallises.

From the solubility let us pass to the spectrum. The hæmoglobin spectra of relatively few forms of life have been studied; but of such as have, no two species yield exactly the same spectrum.

It had been shown indeed by Sorby [4] that the spectra of all hæmoglobins were not the same. The instance which he adduced is the disparity between the hæmoglobin of the snail *Planorbis* and that of vertebrate blood. The following is his statement of the positions of the centres (not necessarily the positions of maximum density) of the bands:

		Centres of bands (Ångström units)	
		α	β
Vertebrate oxyhæmoglobin	...	5810	5450
Planorbis oxyhæmoglobin	...	5780	5425

The position of the α-band differed in the two forms by about 30 Ångström units, and of the β-band by about 25. Gamgee [5] denied this difference. It is only to be supposed that the instruments of former days were too rough for the task of settling the matter. The merest glance with the Hartridge reversion spectroscope, which shows the relative positions of the point of maximum density of the bands, demonstrates the difference between the spectrum of *Planorbis* blood and that of, say, human blood. Twenty-five Ångström units are quite a large disparity with an instrument which will work to about two Ångström units. So far as my own observations go, Sorby was not very wide of the mark.

But Sorby's results lay forgotten, and the question was raised again by Vlès[6], in 1922, who carefully mapped out the spectra of a number of animals, notably *Arenicola* and the horse, finding quite considerable differences.

My own attention was attracted to the matter at the Physiological Congress at Edinburgh in 1923. Wishing to demonstrate a little apparatus for the equilibration of small quantities of blood, I thought it would form a striking demonstration to make some observations with it on the blood of the earthworm. At once, in the Hartridge spectroscope, I saw that the bands were differently placed from those of human hæmoglobin, and also, that they were displaced to a less degree by treatment with carbon monoxide.

Even now work has only commenced on the subject of the exact positions of the spectral bands throughout the animal kingdom; but the following table gives the positions of the α-band of hæmoglobin for a number of animals relatively to that for man[7]. The table also gives data for the α-band of oxyhæmoglobin and of CO-hæmoglobin.

Animal	Position of α-band in Ångström units		Span (S) in Ångström units which separates the α-bands of COHb and O_2Hb
	O_2Hb	COHb	
Man	5769	5709	60
Arenicola (mean)	5751	5697	54
Lumbricus ...	5760	5719	41
Planorbis ...	5751	5707	44
Chironomus ...	5782	5726	56
Pigeon	5767	5709	58
Carp	5767	5715	52
Horse	5769	5707	62
Tortoise	5771	5716	55
Fowl	5774	5717	57
Lizard	5767	5714	53

The question naturally arises: Do the above figures indicate a true specificity, or do they merely signify mixtures of two or three kinds of hæmoglobin in various proportions?

In order to gain some light on this subject samples of hæmoglobin of different spectroscopic constants were partially crystallised (7). It might be supposed that one or other fraction would crystallise out, leaving the rest in the solution, and that, therefore, the residual solution and the redissolved crystals would differ spectroscopically both from the original solution and from one another. The following table gives the "span," i.e. the distance between the α-bands for oxy- and CO-hæmoglobin of various animals before crystallisation and after resolution of the crystals:

Animal	Temp.	Span (Ångström units)	
		Before	After
Rat ...	17° C.	58	58
Horse ...	19° C.	59	59
Rabbit ...	15–16° C.	52	52
Dog ...	15° C.	61·5	61·5

Two interesting cases may be cited, in each of which a couple of specific hæmoglobins may be found within the same animal. The first was carried out by my friend Mr Charles Stockman (7). A leech was starved until its alimentary canal was presumed to be free from blood. It was then given a meal of that material at my own expense, and ten days later it was examined. The blood in the alimentary canal was considerable in amount and was indistinguishable from that in my own vessels; that from the vessels of the leech itself was quite different from either. This was done in the case of two separate leeches.

The second case is more interesting in many ways, one of which is that it has been so productive of future research, being the starting-point of Keilin's (7) researches. The larva of the bot-fly grows within the horse. Its life-history is as follows. The eggs are found on the hair of the horse above the hoof. The horse licks the hair and so ingests the larvæ, which develop in his stomach wall. There the larvæ attain the size of acorns, and within them is found a considerable quantity of hæmoglobin. This hæmoglobin is clearly all manufactured within the horse, but it is quite different from equine hæmoglobin, the bands being nearer to the red in the *Gastrophilus* larva, and the span shorter.

Animal	Position of α-band in Ångström units		Span
	O_2Hb	COHb	
Gastrophilus	5781	5724	57
Horse ...	5772	5710	61

At present we know but little of any classification of the positions of the spectral bands. In so far as there is any phylogenetic arrangement the only things that can be said at present with regard to the α-band of oxyhæmoglobin are: (1) The band is nearest the red in two flies—or rather their larvæ, *Gastrophilus* and *Chironomus*, 5782 A.U. (2) It is nearest the blue in the worms, *Lumbricus* and *Arenicola* [8], and is similarly situated in the mollusc (5760–5745 A.U.). (3) It occupies an intermediate position in the vertebrates (5773–5760 A.U.). What these differences mean when translated into terms of function, or whether they have any meaning, is not known. But though the cause of the difference in span in different animals is unknown, it is likely enough to be important. My reason for saying so is the following:

Already it has been stated that different animals of the same species may have different spans. Within my small experience, that is particularly true of rabbits. When discussing the matter once with Sir Charles Sherrington, he made the suggestion that the span in rabbits differed, not because of any hereditary disparity, but because some rabbits were not in such good health as others. The suggestion would be no less than that the span of a rabbit's blood can change. And this appears to be the case. Litarczek and Stromberger [9], working in the Cambridge laboratory on anæmia, put the matter to the test. They determined the span by the Hartridge reversion spectroscope in the case of six rabbits, while W. H. Forbes determined it for them photographically in the case of one.

The following are the data of the rabbit on whose blood Forbes made the photographic observations; they are compared with those of my own blood, which may serve as a standard since the measurements are in arbitrary units:

	Barcroft blood	Normal rabbit	(Ditto) after treatment
Span in arbitrary units	3·77 (59 A.U.)	3·25	2·62

The rabbits were subject to a certain experimental procedure, the influence of which is obscure, the one important fact being that the span changed, as indeed it has been known to do, without any treatment (Mrs Kerridge).

Reasons will be given later in this chapter for the supposition that the alteration in the span is due to alteration in the globin; they may not be very strong ones, but, if true, surely a remarkable phenomenon confronts us. Why, and how, should the globin of a rabbit's hæmoglobin alter on hæmorrhage? Many answers might be given but they would be mere speculations. Other questions arise, however, which loom distant and large through mists of uncertainty: Is globin merely a sample? Do all the proteins in the body change?

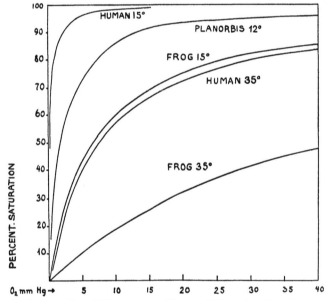

FIG. 8. Oxygen dissociation curves of hæmoglobins of various forms of life at different temperatures.

Let us leave that field for one in which the facts are more concrete. We come to the specificity of hæmoglobin in respect to its affinity for gases. The first workers to draw attention to this phase of the problem were Douglas, Haldane and Haldane (10). In 1912 they showed that if a solution of hæmoglobin made by diluting blood one hundred times with distilled water were exposed to ·093 per cent. CO in air, the hæmoglobin became 67 per cent., or 49 per cent. saturated, according as it was human blood or that of a mouse. No further observation was made on the subject until the oxygen dissociation curve of *Arenicola* was determined, and this appeared to be different from that of human hæmoglobin under similar circumstances, i.e. in a dilute solution of known strength and buffered to a given hydrogen-ion concentration (8).

Since that time the oxygen dissociation curves of hæmoglobins from a number of different species have been investigated, many of them by Maçela and Seliškar (11). They are all different. The difference cannot be stated by a simple constant because it depends upon the temperature. Figs. 8 and 10 show, however, that frog's hæmoglobin holds to its oxygen with much less tenacity than that of some of the low forms of life.

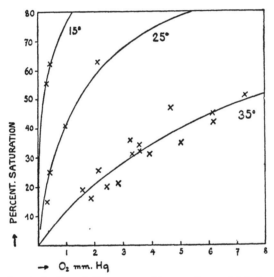

FIG. 9. Approximate O_2 dissociation curve of human hæmoglobin in dilute solution at different temperatures.

The remarkable effect of temperature on the dissociation curve of human hæmoglobin is shown in Fig. 9. The comparison may be expressed thus:

Temp.	Pressure of O_2 at which hæmoglobin is 50 % saturated
15° C.	0·3 mm.
25° C.	1·5 mm.
35° C.	7·5 mm.

In round numbers therefore the pressure corresponding to 50 per cent. saturation rises fivefold for every rise of temperature of 10° C.

For sheep's hæmoglobin in dilute solution, Hartridge and Roughton (12) give the figure 3·8 as representing the temperature coefficient. This, though somewhat less than that of human hæmoglobin, is still very high.

A comparison of the effects of temperature on the hæmoglobins of several forms of life, widely scattered over the animal kingdom, is shown in Fig. 10. The units in which this figure is plotted demand a word of explanation. Take for instance the three points given for human hæmoglobin. They are derived directly from the data given above. The theory need not be discussed at this stage. The pressures for half-saturation are respectively 0·3 mm., 1·5 mm. and 7·5 mm.,

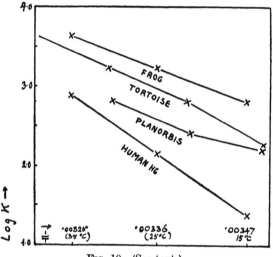

FIG. 10. (See text.)

or 30, 150 and 750 hundredths of a millimetre. The logarithms of these figures are plotted vertically. The horizontal reading is not the absolute temperature but its reciprocal. Thus 25° centigrade is 298° absolute, its reciprocal being ·00336. The effect of temperature then is represented by the slope of the line corresponding to any particular animal. The difference between man and the frog both in the affinity for oxygen and in the effect of temperature on that affinity is easily seen.

In only a very few cases have the curves expressing the equilibrium between reduced hæmoglobin, carboxyhæmoglobin and carbon monoxide been determined, but the following data are forthcoming (8):

Animal	Temperature	Pressure of half-saturation
Man ...	15° C.	$\frac{8}{1000}$ mm.
Arenicola ...	16° C.	$\frac{30}{1000}$ mm. (approximately)

Whilst the latter of these determinations is not very accurate it is at least very different from the former. There is, however, a gas relation about which much more is known than about either that of oxygen or of carbon monoxide to hæmoglobin, namely, the partition of hæmoglobin between the two. It would not be unnatural if the relation of affinity of hæmoglobin for each of the two gases were affected in the same way by whatever influence affects either the one or the other. That indeed is so of hydrogen-ion concentration. An altered hydrogen-ion concentration affects the affinity of hæmoglobin for oxygen, it also affects the affinity of the same substance for CO. The partition coefficient then is not altered. Exposed to a given mixture of oxygen and CO at whatsoever hydrogen-ion concentration, the oxy- and carboxyhæmoglobin will be present in the same proportions. But the cause of the specific differences, whatever it may be, acts differently from hydrogen-ion concentration. That indeed was the essence of the observation of Douglas, Haldane and Haldane on the comparison quoted above of the bloods of man and the mouse respectively.

Not only does the partition coefficient of the reaction

$$COHb + O_2 \rightleftharpoons O_2Hb + CO$$

vary, but the variation seems not to be a function of the affinity of hæmoglobin for either of the two gases concerned.

The reaction equilibrium of the system: oxygen, carbon monoxide, oxyhæmoglobin and carboxyhæmoglobin, may be expressed quantitatively in a very simple way. The quotient of the concentration of CO-hæmoglobin by that of oxyhæmoglobin bears a constant relation to the quotient of the concentration of CO by that of oxygen (using square brackets to denote "the concentration of")

$$\frac{[COHb]}{[O_2Hb]} = K \frac{[CO]}{[O_2]}.$$

Such a relation may of course be plotted graphically if the value of K is known. For man at 15° C. it is about 540[1].

---

[1] This is the relative concentration of the two gases in the solution which corresponds to a figure of 400 for the relative concentration in the atmosphere above the solution.

48 HÆMOGLOBIN

If therefore the carboxy- and oxyhæmoglobin are present in equal amounts, so that

$$\frac{[COHb]}{[O_2Hb]} = 1,$$

the concentration of O_2 will be 540 times that of carbon monoxide.

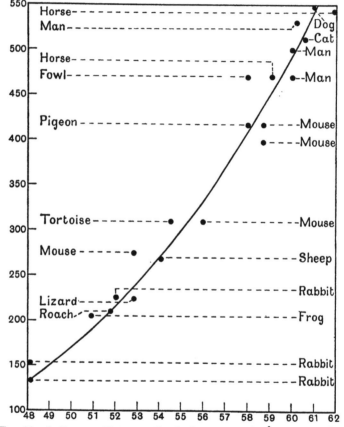

Fig. 11. Ordinate $= K$ (see text); abscissa $=$ span in Ångström units.

The value of K is found to be specific, even individual; not only is it different in the blood of one species from what it is in the blood of another, but it differs even between individuals of the same species.

The same was seen to be true of another relation of hæmoglobin to carbon monoxide and oxygen respectively—namely, the shifting of the a-band in the spectrum. We are now faced with a remarkable relation. The greater the extent by which the a-band of oxyhæmoglobin is shifted by exposure to CO, the greater the value of K in the above equation (7). This is the more remarkable because no relation is known to exist between the absolute positions of the α-band of oxyhæmoglobin and the affinity of hæmoglobin either for oxygen or for carbon monoxide.

The somewhat mysterious relation between the shifting of the α-band of oxyhæmoglobin towards the blue by saturation with CO, and

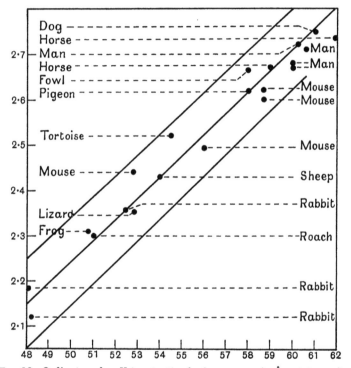

FIG. 12. Ordinate = log K (see text); abscissa = span in Ångström units.

the affinity for CO relative to that for oxygen, is shown in Fig. 11, in which the "span" is plotted against the value of K. The points all have a large experimental error; but the curve bears so logarithmic a character that it seems worth re-plotting it as one in which the "span" is plotted against the logarithm of K. The result is shown in Fig. 12; the outer lines represent the experimental error. No great stress must be laid on the straightness of the central line. It is very short and over so short a range portions of many shallow curves or S-shaped curves might easily appear straight; but it seems difficult to doubt that a relation of some sort exists.

The importance of such a relationship appears when some attempt is made to assign a reason either for the variability of the span, or the variability of K, for if the span and K bear any simple relation to one another it would follow that a cause which alters one alters both.

The most natural opening to the problem of the variation in the span is to ask: Is it due to some disparity in the hæmatins of the various hæmoglobins or to the proteins? To this question an answer can be attempted. By reduction in alkaline solution the globins may be denatured and the corresponding hæmochromogens produced. There is no measurable difference in the positions of the hæmochromogen bands, even though the hæmoglobins from which the hæmochromogens were made differ spectroscopically [7]. Of course if we go into the larger world of hæmochromogens made by the attachment of pyridine, nicotine, etc. to hæmatin we do get differences, the hæmochromogen bands are shifted a little one way or the other, but the spectra of hæmochromogens built on a basis of denatured globin are all the same [13]. It would appear therefore that the denaturation of the globin reduced all hæmoglobin spectra to a common level, and that would go to show that the specific differences in the spectra of different vertebrate bloods found an explanation in the properties of the undenatured globin present.

If it be then that the span is related to the gas-bearing properties of hæmoglobin we are brought to believe that the fine adjustment, so far as these properties are concerned, rests in the globin portion of the molecule, and that human blood has a different affinity for oxygen to frog's blood, not because its hæmoglobin is built upon a different basis of porphyrin, but because its porphyrin is attached to a different globin. And what is true of the affinity for oxygen would be true of the temperature coefficient of the same, and this truth would confer on globin a definite rôle in the evolution of the animal kingdom.

REFERENCES

(1) REICHERT AND BROWN. *The Crystallography of Hæmoglobins.* 1909.

(2) LANDSTEINER AND HEIDELBERGER. *Journ. Gen. Physiol.* VI. 131. 1923.

(3) FERRY. *Journ. Biol. Chem.* LVII. 819. 1923.

(4) SORBY. *Quart. Journ. Micr. Sci.* XVI. 76. 1876.

(5) GAMGEE. *Physiological Chemistry of the Animal Body,* vol. I. chap. II. p. 131. 1880.

(6) VLÈS. *Arch. Phys. Biol.* II. 21. 1922.

(7) ANSON, BARCROFT, MIRSKY AND OINUMA. *Proc. Roy. Soc.* B. XCVII. 61. 1925.

(8) BARCROFT, J. AND BARCROFT, H. *Proc. Roy. Soc.* B. XCVI. 28. 1924.

(9) LITARCZEK AND STROMBERGER. In press.

(10) DOUGLAS, HALDANE, J. S. AND HALDANE, J. B. S. *Journ. Physiol.* XLIV. 275. 1912.

(11) MAÇELA AND SELIŠKAR. *Journ. Physiol.* LX. 428. 1925.

(12) HARTRIDGE AND ROUGHTON. *Proc. Roy. Soc.* A. CIV. 395. 1923.

(13) ANSON AND MIRSKY. *Journ. Physiol.* LX. 50. 1925.

CHAPTER VI

SPECIFIC OXYGEN CAPACITY

THE specific oxygen capacity is the relation of the oxygen to the iron in hæmoglobin. Its interest lay at first in its relation to the question of whether or no there was more than one kind of hæmoglobin. On other grounds it is agreed that there are innumerable kinds of hæmoglobin, the protein in each being specific to the organism. When I wrote the original edition of *The Respiratory Function of the Blood*, the specific oxygen capacity of hæmoglobin was again on the *tapis*. The question then was: Is oxygen united chemically to hæmoglobin or is the union one of adsorption? Here again it seems to me that opinion has crystallised. In this country, as far as I know, Bayliss[1] was the last writer who sympathised with the view that oxyhæmoglobin was purely an adsorptive compound. I do not know of any such in America and, in Europe, if there are they, like Bayliss, are persons whose interest is rather in adsorption than in hæmoglobin.

We have now reached a yet higher plane. The question in front of us is as follows: When hæmoglobin is present, to what extent are other iron-containing bodies present also? We have stated the view that hæmoglobin is only maintained *in statu quo* as part of a mass action which involves hæmochromogen and that hæmochromogen itself only exists in the presence of reduced hæmatin[2]. Of these three substances, hæmoglobin, hæmochromogen and reduced hæmatin, only one, hæmoglobin, contains oxygen which can be abstracted in the free state by ferricyanide or by a vacuum, whilst all three contain iron. It follows, therefore, that more iron must be present than is equivalent to the oxygen. The question is: How much more iron? If the ratio of iron to oxygen is not considerably greater than 56 grams of iron to every 32 of oxygen, the hæmoglobin phase of the reaction must be almost complete and the quantities of hæmochromogen and hæmatin negligible.

Conant and Scott suggest, on the other hand, that while most of the oxygen is present in chemical combination, an additional portion is adsorbed; if so there should be more than 32 grams of oxygen to 56 of iron in blood.

In the present state of our knowledge it is by no means a foregone conclusion that the desirable relationship which we have described should exist. Presumably it depends upon a correspondence between the properties of the particular globin which is present in the hæmoglobin and the conditions which are to be found in the blood; and it seems possible that some slight change in the nature of the globin might produce a hæmochromogen which was much less likely than that of the normal body to go completely to hæmoglobin. There would be an appreciable quantity of iron in excess of oxygen. If, on the other hand, the excess of iron is not measurable, it follows that the background of iron-containing bodies is inappreciable in mass and is only of theoretical interest.

Much laborious work has been done on the determination of the "specific oxygen capacity" of hæmoglobin. Suppose, for instance, that it appears as the result of analysis that 401 cubic centimetres of oxygen correspond invariably to a gram of iron, it would follow that hæmoglobin obeyed the law of definite proportions so far as oxygen and iron were concerned, and also that it obeyed the law of combination in simple proportions. For expressing this ratio of the iron to the oxygen by weight every 56 grams of iron would correspond to 32 grams of oxygen. In other words the oxygen and the iron would be united in the proportion of one atom of iron to two of oxygen.

The following table will, however, show that the history of the subject provides us with but scanty hope of reaching this ideal.

Observer	Animal	Number of cases	Extreme figures	Mean specific oxygen capacity
Bohr [3]	Dog	22	328–468	375
Tobiesen [4]	Dog and calf	17	378–429	388
Abrahamsen [5] ...	Ox	32	301–391	351
„	Pig	5	284–401	341
Bohr [6]	Horse	9	379–426	411
Bornstein and Müller [7]	Cat	5	372–403	401
Masing and Siebeck [8]	Man, ox, rabbit	—	—	397
Butterfield [9]	Ox	3	389–395	397
„	Man	—	—	391
„	Man (diseased)	11	384–409	399

The discrepancies between the various analyses amount in some cases to one-third of the whole quantity of oxygen measured, and some little consideration must be given to their interpretation. It will be noted that the figures are spread both above and below 401, the average being usually rather below that figure.

There were two schools of thought with regard to these figures when they were published. Of these the first taught that the sources of analytical error were so great as to make more accurate analysis impossible, whilst the second, represented chiefly by the late Prof. Christian Bohr [10] of Copenhagen, frankly admitted that the want of uniformity was so great as to render untenable the idea of hæmoglobin as a single substance. He explained the divergences which we have noted as being due to a mixture of four substances which he called α-, β-, γ-, and δ-hæmoglobins, each with a different oxygen capacity from the others.

To the schools mentioned a third was added by Wolfgang Ostwald, which taught that the combination of oxygen and hæmoglobin was not in the old-fashioned sense a chemical combination, but a manifestation of the physical phenomenon known as adsorption, and that it therefore depended upon electric charges on the molecules of the oxygen and hæmoglobin. The amount and nature of the charges present might be supposed to vary, and, in so doing, affect the amount of oxygen with which a given quantity of iron would unite.

Lastly there is the school of thought now just opening which regards the hæmoglobin molecule not as something static but rather as a dynamic system and one which involves the presence of other iron-containing bodies. To what extent is the proportion which they bear to hæmoglobin constant?

Since Bohr's time, partly on account of the improvements in the analytical methods both for oxygen and iron, and partly on account of the increased importance of the subject, it became more and more desirable that some reinvestigation, by direct methods, of the specific oxygen capacity of hæmoglobin, should take place. I mean by direct methods those in which the oxygen was measured as such and the iron as a salt of that metal, as opposed to indirect spectrophotometric methods, which have given uniform and apparently excellent results in the hands of Butterfield. This investigation was undertaken by Peters[1] [11]; for the purpose of estimating the oxygen he used the differential method of blood-gas analysis, based upon the observation of Haldane that oxygen is eliminated from hæmoglobin quantitatively by potassium ferricyanide [12].

[1] Now Professor of Biochemistry at Oxford.

The theoretical accuracy of the ferricyanide method was regarded at that time as proved by the researches of Haldane, confirmed by those of Franz Müller in Berlin [13]. Certainly these authors proved it not to be grossly inaccurate. Recent research has shown a certain source of error in its use for the determination of the oxygen in blood [14]. The fats in the plasma react with the ferricyanide and use up some oxygen in the process. This effect in normal blood is very slow, hence in a method as rapid as the differential method of oxygen estimation which Peters used, this error is scarcely perceptible, though in the case of anæmic and consequently lipæmic animals it becomes very appreciable. By using the differential method Peters had no difficulty in doing half a dozen determinations with as many cubic centimetres of blood in two hours. Even had Peters used blood—not a suspension of corpuscles—he would have been at a great advantage as compared with his predecessors, whose individual analyses, if theoretically somewhat more accurate, extended over two or three days, and entailed the use of large quantities of hæmoglobin. It was impossible in their case to obtain large numbers of analyses from which the errors could be eliminated to some extent by statistical treatment.

In estimating the iron by titration with titanium advantage was taken of new methods of analysis which were much simpler and more accurate than the older permanganate titrations.

The theory of the titanium method of estimating iron is represented by the following equation:

$$TiCl_3 + FeCl_3 = TiCl_4 + FeCl_2.$$

The method has this great advantage over that of titration with potassium permanganate, that it is not vitiated by the presence of chlorides.

In practice defibrinated blood was centrifugalised, the corpuscles washed twice in isotonic salt solution and as much as possible of the fluid removed. The cream of corpuscles was laked by twice its volume of dilute ammonia (4 c.c. of strong ammonia per litre). This solution, which we shall call solution A, was centrifugalised again to rid it of any corpuscles which did not lake and of other debris. Portions of it were then measured out of the same burette both for the iron estimations and for the oxygen analyses. For the former 50 c.c. of the solution were evaporated in a platinum crucible and carefully "ashed." It was at this point that the nicety of the determinations really entered, if accurate results were to be obtained. The "ashing" must take place at a temperature which is neither too hot nor too cold. It is best carried out in a muffle furnace. To quote Peters: "If the carbon is not completely burned away iron will still remain, which cannot be removed by boiling with acids; whereas, on the other hand, if the ash is heated to a high temperature the iron becomes insoluble. In both cases there will be a loss of iron." After the "ashing" is complete the iron is dissolved in strong hydrochloric acid, and a trace of hydrogen peroxide is added to ensure the complete oxidation of the iron. The excess of hydrogen peroxide is subsequently boiled off, and the titration with titanous chloride is made, potassium sulphocyanide being used as an indicator.

Some idea of the scale on which Peters' experiments were conducted may be gleaned from an account of a single experiment. In addition to making two analyses of iron such as have just been described, he made from the same solution, run from the same burette, sixteen oxygen estimations. These were divided into four groups: the average of each group was taken and also the mean of these four averages. The greatest error which entered into Peters' blood-gas analysis was doubtless in the measurement of 3 c.c. of fluid from an ordinary 50 c.c. burette, the meniscus in the case of hæmoglobin solution being none too well defined. This error, serious though it appears, is discounted by the fact that the sixteen samples for analysis were run consecutively out of the burette. There may be a certain ruggedness in the individual figures, but the averages of the groups of four are very close to one another, since a positive error in one sample entails an equal negative error in the next: in the aggregate 48 c.c. used there is no appreciable error as compared with the 50 c.c. used by the iron analysis.

Peters' figures for the oxygen are as follows:

Oxygen in 3 c.c. of solution A in c.c.

	Group I	Group II	Group III	Group IV
	·3667	·3667	·3576	·3527
	·3449	·3374	·3640	·3510
	·3482	·3439	·3638	·3614
	·3455	·3517	·3455	·3537
Total ...	1·4053	1·3997	1·4309	1·4188
Mean ...	·3513	·3499	·3577	·3547

Taking the average of these four means we get

·3513
·3499
·3577
·3547

Total ... 1·4136
Mean ... ·3534 c.c.

When it is remembered that the whole of these operations, both iron analyses and gas analyses, could be carried through successfully in a day, it will be clear what an advance Peters made by the use of the then modern technique, both as regards the concordance of his figures, and the certainty with which he has been able to put them forward. His figures for the volume of oxygen per gram of iron are as follows:

Ox ...	...	...	394, 401, 399
Sheep	...	...	387, 384
Pig ...	...	...	388
Dog	...	...	384
	Average	...	391

It is not very easy to discern the processes by which conviction grows in the mind; probably the mere inspection of the figures given is sufficient to convince the reader that so far as the relation of the respiratory oxygen to the iron of hæmoglobin is concerned, these quantities are related in the proportions of two atoms of oxygen to one of iron. To me, who had the privilege of seeing Peters' work from week to week, conviction came in a slightly different way; it developed as it were like the image on a photographic plate. As one experimental difficulty after another was overcome, as one source of error after another was weeded out, as the worker himself developed in skill and in capacity, just so surely did the results which he obtained approach the theoretical figure with greater certainty until, at the end, when all the difficulties had been overcome, and when Peters himself had attained to the rank of a first-rate exponent of the technique, I arrived at a stage of conviction in which I never doubted, when he undertook an experiment, that the result would be between 385 and 405. Perhaps there could be no surer proof that all thought of the wide differences between different kinds of hæmoglobin, alleged to exist by Bohr and others, had passed out of our horizon than the fact of our almost laughable concern at the end as to why the average figure was 391 and not 401. We in the laboratory thought, perhaps, that Peters did not perform sufficient experiments to obtain a true average, or that some trace of methæmoglobin was always present, or that some trifling error was always present in the standardisation of the apparatus used.

A very careful recalibration of the apparatus by another method was undertaken by Burn[15], who obtained a result 2·5 per cent. higher than that given by the method which Peters used.

Nowadays neither the method used by Peters nor that used by Burn would be employed, the calibration of the apparatus being carried out by some form of the method described by Hoffmann [16]. There is of course quite a literature on the subject as the differential gas apparatus has come into general use for many types of respiratory work. A very convenient method of calibration is that described by Münzer and Neumann [17], and quoted in Ludwig Pincussen's book [18], but that is a digression. Looking back from the distance of fifteen years there are several points which deserve a word of comment.

(1) By separating the corpuscles from the plasma and discarding the latter, Peters' results stand free of the principal criticism to which the use of ferricyanide in the differential apparatus has been subjected, namely, that of a too low oxygen reading caused by auto-oxidation of the ferricyanide by the lipoids in the plasma.

(2) Peters' figures are certainly not above 401. Bayliss [19] put forward the suggestion that the hæmoglobin in these and similar experiments was not really saturated, and that if exposed to a greater concentration of oxygen, it would unite with more of that gas.

Subsequent work has failed to bear out Bayliss' contention. I tested the matter with the following result [19]. I exposed blood to a gaseous mixture of 85 per cent. oxygen and 15 per cent. nitrogen, and found the following percentage degrees of saturation as compared with that regarded as complete: 102, 99, 98 and 97 in four experiments. These values were corrected for the gas physically dissolved, and pointed to a true saturation point.

W. E. L. Brown [20] also approached it in another way; he argued thus. Carbon monoxide has, say, 250 times the affinity for hæmoglobin that oxygen has (more or less according to the hæmoglobin in question). An exposure to 1 atmosphere of CO should then saturate the hæmoglobin to the same degree as exposure to 250 atmospheres of oxgyen, or exposure to $\frac{1}{5}$ atmosphere of CO should have an effect quantitatively equal to 250 atmospheres of air. Brown, however, found that when blood which had been equilibrated with oxygen in air was exposed to carbon monoxide, the quantity of carbon monoxide taken up was neither greater nor less than that of the oxygen which was given out. It would appear then that aerated blood did not fall short of saturation with oxygen, by any measurable quantity. Peters' results are justified of criticism on that point.

(3) Granting that his results are not above 401, are they below it? and if so, why? Already it has been stated (a) that as given by Peters

himself, the average figure came to 391; (*b*) that on a recalibration by Burn it came to 401; (*c*) that better methods of calibration now exist; but the particular apparatus used by Peters has long since vanished, even the type is no longer made.

There remains the possibility therefore that some 2 per cent. of the iron present was contained in substances which do not yield their oxygen to ferricyanide.

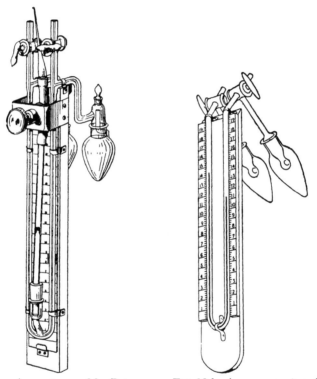

FIG. 13 *a*. Apparatus used by Peters.   FIG. 13 *b*. A more recent model.

If one enquires what these substances may be, first there is methæmoglobin. Two parts of methæmoglobin are not very easy to detect in one hundred parts of oxyhæmoglobin. The spectrum would not show them and it would require very accurate analytical methods to do so.

The second substance, known as "inactive hæmoglobin," is to be considered. Could 2 per cent. of the hæmoglobin have been in the inactive state? Peters unconsciously reduced his problem to its simplest terms by using hæmoglobin made directly from blood without any crystallisation previous to his determinations. In this way he avoided the contamination of the pigment with a substance, as yet little studied, namely, "inactive hæmoglobin." This substance has been handled by most workers interested in blood pigments, the clearest statement of its properties coming from the Rockefeller Institute. My own acquaintance with it recalls an interesting reminiscence. When A. V. Hill sat for his final examination in Cambridge, I had the experience of examining him, and I set this question in the practical examination: "Prepare a 5 per cent. solution of hæmoglobin." My idea was that, starting with blood, the candidates should measure the oxygen capacity, assume that each cubic centimetre of oxygen which they obtained represented $1/1\cdot34$ grams of hæmoglobin and, having found the percentage of hæmoglobin present (presumably about 15 per cent.), dilute the blood with water till it became 5 per cent. Incidentally the blood would be laked and the hæmoglobin thrown into solution. Hill, however, proceeded otherwise. He made the crystals, dried and weighed them and then dissolved up five grams of the weighed crystals in water. The colour of the final solution did not commend itself to me, and wishing to ascertain the amount of methæmoglobin which it contained I endeavoured to test its oxygen capacity with ferricyanide. To my great surprise it yielded no oxygen: at the same time its spectrum, on a casual examination, was that of oxyhæmoglobin. Bayliss [21], I know, also observed a similar phenomenon.

The following is the statement made on the subject by Van Slyke, Hastings, Heidelberger and Neill [22]:

> If dried, even at high vacuum and in the cold, hæmoglobin is almost completely inactivated, although in solubility and colour it still resembles oxyhæmoglobin. Slow loss of activity occurs even while standing in solution. The maximum loss in our preparations was one-fifth of the theoretical oxygen capacity.

The presence of this tautomeric form may have had something to do with the anomalous results obtained by Bohr, his instinct would have been to purify his hæmoglobin to the maximum extent possible by crystallisation. It is one of the ironies of hæmoglobin that the greater the pains at which you are to make it pure the greater is the extent to which you are likely to contaminate it by the formation of the "inactive" variety.

Whether inactive hæmoglobin occurs in nature we do not know. obviously it was not present in more than the most trifling quantities in the bloods which were investigated by Peters, though it may have been present to the extent of 1 or 2 per cent. of the whole hæmoglobin analysed; these experiments, however, only covered a very limited range of the animal kingdom and took no account of pathological cases. Curious things can occur. I once killed a rat which had brown blood, yet a casual observation with the spectroscope failed to reveal the cause.

Recent research has revealed another substance—is it another substance? or is it the same under another name?—that substance is variously called kathæmoglobin or parahæmatin. It was described by Arnold [23] and v. Klaveren [24], and has been investigated recently by Keilin [25]. Briefly, when hæmochromogen is oxidised within very narrow limits of hydrogen-ion concentration, near neutrality, parahæmatin is formed. The protein does not split off from the hæmatin, as according to them it does if the solution is alkaline, but remains attached to it. The result is a substance possessing a spectrum which bears a superficial resemblance to oxyhæmoglobin, but which does not yield up its oxygen to potassium ferricyanide or to a vacuum. Whether parahæmatin and inactive hæmoglobin are the same thing, or are different things, remains to be seen. If, however, Peters' estimate of the specific oxygen capacity of hæmoglobin was 2 per cent. too low the presence of parahæmatin must be included among the possible causes.

In no case, however, is there reason to doubt that the iron and the oxygen in hæmoglobin are united in the proportions of two atoms of detachable oxygen to one of iron.

REFERENCES

(1) BAYLISS. *Principles of General Physiology*, chap. XXI. 2nd ed. 1918.

(2) ANSON AND MIRSKY. *Journ. Physiol.* LX. 50. 1925.

(3) BOHR. *Skand. Arch. f. Physiol.* III. 101. 1892.

(4) TOBIESEN. *Skand. Arch. f. Physiol.* VI. 273. 1895.

(5) ABRAHAMSEN. *Über den Sauerstoff des Blutes*, 47. Kopenhagen, 1893.

(6) BOHR. For a full discussion *vide* Nagel's *Handbuch*, I. 93. 1909.

(7) BORNSTEIN AND MÜLLER. *Arch. f. Anat. u. Physiol.* p. 470. 1907.

(8) MASING AND SIEBECK. *Deut. Arch. für Klin. Med.* XCVIII. 123. 1909; XCIX. 130. 1910.

(9) BUTTERFIELD. *Zeitsch. Physiol. Chem.* XLII. 143. 1909.

(10) BOHR. *Skand. Arch. f. Physiol.* III. 76. 1892.

(11) PETERS. *Journ. Physiol.* XLIV. 131. 1912.

(12) HALDANE. *Journ. Physiol.* XXII. 298. 1898; XXV. 295. 1900.

(13) MÜLLER, FRANZ. *Pflüger's Archiv,* CIII. 541. 1904.

(14) LITARCZEK. *Journ. Physiol.* 1926. In press.

(15) BARCROFT AND BURN. *Journ. Physiol.* XLV. 493. 1913.

(16) HOFFMANN. *Journ. Physiol.* XLVII. 272. 1913–1914.

(17) MÜNZER AND NEUMANN. *Biochem. Zeitsch.* LXXXI. 319. 1917.

(18) PINCUSSEN, LUDWIG. *Mikromethodik.*

(19) BAYLISS. *Principles of General Physiology,* chap. XXI. p. 614. 1924.

(20) BROWN, W. E. L. *Nature,* III. 881. 1923.

(21) BAYLISS. From conversation.

(22) VAN SLYKE, HASTINGS, HEIDELBERGER AND NEILL. *Journ. Biol. Chem.* LIV. 481. 1922.

(23) ARNOLD. *Zeitsch. Physiol. Chem.* XXIX. 78. 1900.

(24) v. KLAVEREN. *Zeitsch. Physiol. Chem.* XXXIII. 293. 1901.

(25) KEILIN. *Proc. Roy. Soc.* B. c. 130. 1926.

CHAPTER VII

THE MANUFACTURE OF HÆMOGLOBIN

THE specific oxygen capacity of hæmoglobin can be determined with accuracy on "whole blood" because there is in that fluid no other substance which contains an appreciable quantity of iron. If the properties of the pigment are to be examined in detail it is necessary to have some definite ideas about the preparation of the pigment in a state of purity. It is at this point that hæmoglobin begins to present those elusive qualities which conspire to make it "perhaps the most interesting substance in the world." Could we, once and for all, give a complete statement of why hæmoglobin on all occasions acts as it does, we should have made strides with seven league boots through the realm of colloid chemistry, and more than that—it is possible that we should have shortened to an appreciable extent the journey which must be traversed before we obtain any true insight into the difference between living and dead matter.

The classical method for the preparation of hæmoglobin is somewhat as follows. You obtain blood from some animal the hæmoglobin of which crystallises out with ease. Here then is a crop of problems as yet quite unsolved: Why does the blood of some animals crystallise more readily than that of others? On what property of the hæmoglobin does its tendency to form crystals depend? Why are the crystals from the bloods of different animals, and even from the blood of the same animal, of different forms? We attribute the difference to the globin, and for the present we must let the matter pass with the statement that the blood of the rat crystallises with great ease, e.g. on the addition of distilled water, and that the horse and dog are the animals from which it is most easy to obtain hæmoglobin crystals in bulk. Indeed crystals of hæmoglobin may be prepared from horse blood by a process no more elaborate than that of passing the blood through a Sharpless separator (1) reputed to revolve at 17,000 revolutions per minute; this procedure we have seen in Prof. Laurence J. Henderson's laboratory. To return to the classical method, starting with the blood of the horse, or if such cannot be obtained then the blood of the dog—but in no wise using the blood of the ox, sheep or pig, for they do not readily crystallise—

you concentrate the corpuscles into a creamy mass in a centrifuge, draw off the plasma, wash the corpuscles two or three times with saline, then add sufficient alcohol (or ether) to lake the blood and throw down the crystals. Having obtained the crystals you wash them with ice-cold water on a porous plate, you then dry them, put them in a bottle which you label "hæmoglobin," and there they are. You may have an easy mind so long as you refrain from asking yourself the following question: "What relation does the brown powder in the bottle bear to the pigment which existed in the corpuscles?"

In many ways we have more to learn about the condition of hæmoglobin in the interior of the corpuscles than was supposed twenty or thirty years ago; nevertheless this much may be said upon the chemical side, hæmoglobin behaves in some ways like an acid, in others like an alkali. For instance it unites with such dyes as stain oxyphil granules indicating that it has certain basic properties. The colour which it assumes when stained with eosin for example depends rather upon the number than upon the strength of such affinities, and there is no reason for connecting them particularly with the hæmatin rather than the protein part of the molecule. In the main, however, hæmoglobin must be regarded as an acid, and oxyhæmoglobin as a stronger acid than reduced hæmoglobin. In the corpuscle, the reaction of which is on the alkaline side of neutral, it may be supposed that we have a salt of the acid, this salt being the sodium, or potassium salt, according to the animal concerned; whilst in some animals there will be a mixture of the two. In oxygenated blood corpuscles, therefore, the interiors of which are buffered, probably the hæmoglobin will be present to some extent as the acid, but principally as the sodium or potassium salt and perhaps as a mixture of the two.

To what extent does the above method tend to preserve these relationships? It is obvious that the mere laking of the corpuscles and setting free of the pigment mixes the bases of the interior of the corpuscle with those of the exterior, and therefore the base present in the crystals may be largely that of the fluid in which the corpuscles were suspended. The cure would seem to be that in washing the corpuscles the fluid used should not be the ordinary physiological saline, but a saline made up on a basis of sodium chloride, bicarbonate, etc., if the corpuscles are such as contain sodium, whilst if the corpuscles contain potassium the saline should contain potassium salt. A greater source of solicitude is the advisability of using alcohol or ether at all.

So far as I can appraise the motives of those who have concerned themselves much with the manufacture of hæmoglobin, I discern two distinct points of view, which I may describe as the chemical and the biological. In the end of course they meet, but in essence the chemist wishes to obtain the material in some form in which he can describe it exactly, and be sure that successive samples which he may obtain are identical in composition. To this end the high road is crystallisation. That reagents such as alcohol or ether should be used in the manufacture of the crystals is a small matter, the danger of using them is that the crystal produced may be different from the hæmoglobin as it exists in blood—that is relatively trifling, the important point is that you do get a crystal—a thing which can be washed, which has a definite shape, whose angles are of definite size. This, from the chemist's point of view, is something from which a start can be made. If a stable standard solution of such crystals can be obtained and the properties of such a standard solution described, the worker may proceed to compare it with hæmoglobin as found in blood.

I will describe, then, some methods which have been used for the preparation of hæmoglobin. They do not include various "salting out methods" which the reader can easily find in books of reference.

Of the more modern methods the first to which reference may be made is that of Christian Bohr[2]. It was essentially the procedure adopted by Roberts and myself[3] in 1909:

The solution of hæmoglobin was made as follows: Dog's blood, freshly drawn, was whipped, centrifugalised, and the serum drawn off, Ringer's fluid was then added, to make up to the original bulk, and the corpuscles shaken up. The corpuscles were given three washings with Ringer's fluid in all and then ether added and the mass of corpuscles stirred until a crystalline paste was obtained; this was allowed to stand in the cold over night. The etherial mass was then warmed up to 40° and centrifugalised in warm tubes. The supernatant fluid and the upper portion of the crystalline layer were discarded, the lower portion was slowly dissolved, with constant shaking, in distilled water at 40° until the etherial smell had disappeared and only the characteristic smell proper to dog's blood remained. The solution so prepared was filtered through several layers of filter paper on a Nutsche filter and divided into two portions A and B. Portion A was freed from salts as far as possible by dialysis. The essential difficulty about this operation arose from the time which it took, seeing that there must be no bacterial action in the solution. The following course was adopted. A stoppered glass cylinder of about 10 inches in height and 3 inches in diameter was employed for the dialysis. It was thoroughly rinsed with formalin and the formalin removed by repeated washings with boiled distilled water. The hæmoglobin solution was placed in a parchment tube of the ordinary form. This tube was suspended in boiled distilled water in the glass cylinder. The tube, like the cylinder, was rendered aseptic with formalin and similarly washed. The dialysis was allowed to proceed for 2 days during which time the cylinder stood in ice. The water was changed at intervals of a few hours during the day-time. The earlier samples of water which had been used for the dialysis gave a precipitate when tested with silver nitrate, the later ones did not. At the end the hæmoglobin solution was without odour of any kind. Clearly then the cause of its original odour, as well as all suspicion of formalin, had disappeared.

During the dialysis the hæmoglobin solution became considerably diluted and at the end it gave a reading of approximately 30 with Haldane's standard hæmoglobino-meter. It was necessary therefore to concentrate it. This was done by distillation over a water bath at 40° in an ordinary distillation flask fitted to a condenser. The condenser was surrounded by ice; the whole was kept vacuous by the action of a Tœpler pump fitted with a drying chamber which contained sulphuric acid. The concentration was allowed to proceed until the hæmoglobin solution gave a reading of 70 on the hæmoglobinometer—which was identical with that of portion B.

Portion B was kept in ice during the dialysis of A. To start with it had a hæmo-globin value of 85, and before use it was filtered through a new Berkefeld filter which reduced its hæmoglobin value to 70.

The solutions used subsequently by Barcroft and Hill [4] were made without ether or alcohol. The corpuscles were centrifuged and washed in the manner described above. The apparatus used for dialysis was as described, but the mass of washed corpuscles, not that of crystals, was put straight into the dialyser. The assumption was that as the salts dialysed out the corpuscles burst and hæmoglobin was set free. That this must have been so to a large extent is clear from the fact that there were often considerable masses of hæmoglobin crystals in the bottom of the dialyser, the solution apparently becoming super-saturated. One point may be noted here, namely, that the solutions made in this way never filtered so easily as those made from the resolution of the crystals.

Three other methods of obtaining hæmoglobin crystals on a con-siderable scale may be mentioned. Each of them has considerable merits; they are (1) the method of Dudley and Evans [5], (2) that of Heidelberger [6], and (3) that of Parsons.

(1) The method of Dudley and Evans depends upon the fact that oxyhæmoglobin is less soluble than reduced hæmoglobin. If therefore a saturated solution of reduced hæmoglobin be oxidised, the crystals of oxyhæmoglobin will separate out.

In the application of the method horse corpuscles were washed by centrifugalisation until the washings were free from protein and dialysed in collodion sacs against distilled water under the osmotic pressure of the hæmoglobin itself. In the course of the dialysis the corpuscles were laked and the hæmoglobin became reduced. The thick syrup remaining was then removed, quickly centrifuged to remove the debris and then transferred to a saturator and aerated by rotation when crystals of oxyhæmoglobin separated out. These were purified by centrifuging off the mother liquor, adding distilled water and placing in a vacuum, when the crystals went into solution. These could be thrown out again by re-oxidation. At each resolution, however, a certain amount of insoluble brown material remained and had to be removed by the centrifugal machine.

(2) Heidelberger's method. I am indebted to Dr Michael Heidelberger for the following notes:

The method now proposed depends upon observations that suspensions of washed dog or horse red cells crystallise rapidly and almost completely in the presence of toluene when saturated with carbon dioxide and oxygen, and that the resulting oxyhæmoglobin may be recrystallised by solution with the aid of sodium carbonate and reprecipitation with carbon dioxide.

The use of toluene was found to hasten markedly the crystallisation of the oxyhæmoglobin in the corpuscles owing to its disintegrating effect on the cells themselves. While its hæmolytic action is slower than that of ether, its use obviates the chief disadvantages of the latter, namely, solubility in water, and the presence of peroxides and other reactive substances which may alter oxyhæmoglobin.

The carbon dioxide shifts the reaction in the acid direction past the isoelectric point of oxyhæmoglobin, so that the crystals obtained are oxyhæmoglobin uncombined with alkali. By thus promoting the crystallisation of the oxyhæmoglobin the acidification also aids in the original disintegration of the corpuscles. Saturation with pure carbon dioxide would drive oxygen out of the solution and change the oxyhæmoglobin to the reduced form, which is too soluble to crystallise readily. In order to obviate this difficulty, one part of oxygen is mixed in a cylinder with four of carbon dioxide for the saturation. Such a mixture may be passed through oxyhæmoglobin solutions indefinitely without reduction.

Removal of the salts is accomplished by the simplified form of pressure dialysis suggested by Adair, Barcroft and Bock[7], *after* the desired number of recrystallisations has been carried out. Two recrystallisations have been deemed sufficient in this laboratory, but for many purposes the oxyhæmoglobin will undoubtedly be found pure enough after the first recrystallisation. On the other hand, the losses involved in each recrystallisation, while appreciable, are not sufficiently large to preclude three or even four recrystallisations.

Three precautions have been found essential: 1. All operations are carried out in the cold, centrifugation of the solutions being an exception if a centrifuge in a cold room is not available. 2. The oxyhæmoglobin is not allowed to become dry, owing to the resultant change, noted by Bohr[2], into a modification in which the oxygen is not reactive. 3. During the various manipulations on the acid side of the isoelectric point, before the final dialysis, care is taken to have an excess of carbon dioxide constantly present. If the carbon dioxide tension is permitted to fall, part of the oxyhæmoglobin is redissolved as alkali salt.

The purity of the oxyhæmoglobin obtained by the present method has been controlled by a determination of the ratio of the oxyhæmoglobin present, as determined by Van Slyke and Stadie's procedure (8), to the total hæmoglobin pigments present, determined as cyanhæmoglobin by Stadie's method (9)...preparations of 96 to 100 per cent. of the theoretical oxygen capacity were obtained. The relative freedom of the product from salts was controlled by conductivity measurements of saturated aqueous solutions.

(3) Parsons has very kindly given me a description of his method in the following words:

Starting with the observation that a frozen solution of hæmoglobin consists of a mixture of hæmoglobin crystals and ice crystals, we conceived the idea that if a solution of hæmoglobin were centrifuged while it was being frozen the crystals of ice and hæmoglobin would be separated and the latter would collect at the bottom of the containing tube. We soon proved that this separation does in fact take place under these circumstances, but found the method very difficult to apply as even when the centrifuge was installed in a refrigerating chamber it was very difficult to cool it at a rate sufficient to counterbalance its own rate of production of heat by friction. We therefore later adopted the simpler converse process of centrifuging a frozen hæmoglobin solution while it was allowed to thaw, and in this way obtained a somewhat slower but easier method of concentrating and crystallising the pigment. We find that Offringa (10) had previously observed the crystallisation of horse hæmoglobin during the centrifuging of its frozen solution, but we find further that this process can be used for the crystallisation of the more soluble hæmoglobins such as those of ox and sheep (so that it possesses the great advantage that ordinary slaughterhouse blood can be used for the preparation), and that it can also be used for the crystallisation of the corresponding "reduced" CO- and methæmoglobins of these animals, and for the concentration of hæmocyanin and similar animal pigments. The practical details of the method may be stated quite briefly. The corpuscles are freed from serum proteins by repeated washings in the centrifuge with 1 per cent. sodium chloride solution (which, being slightly hypertonic, causes shrinkage and better settlement). The corpuscle mass, sucked as free as possible from salt solution, is then laked by freezing and thawing repeated twice or three times if necessary. The resulting liquid is placed in a bottle and the stromata are removed from it by vigorous shaking with about 1/10 of its volume of well-washed asbestos pulp for 2 to 3 hours. According to a suggestion made by Bayliss the gradual removal of the stromata on to the surface of the asbestos can be followed by observing the gradual decrease of the viscosity of the solution. The asbestos is removed by centrifuging and the solution of hæmoglobin is divided among the centrifuge tubes which, after balancing, are placed in the refrigerator or freezing mixture in order that their contents may freeze. The freezing should be carried out at a temperature in the neighbourhood of − 5° to − 7° C., i.e. well above − 22° C., which is the cryohydric point at which crystals of solid sodium chloride separate out. When the freezing is complete the tubes are placed in the machine and rotated at a speed of at least 4000 revolutions per minute until complete thawing has taken place. With tubes holding about 120 c.c. each this takes about 20 to 30 minutes under ordinary conditions. This freezing and centrifuging are then repeated some five to six times, by which time the upper layers of the liquid in the tubes will be found to be practically colourless while the hæmoglobin will have crystallised out at the botton. Care must of course be taken not to disturb the layers of liquid during the manipulations. When sufficient crystals have been collected in this way the upper liquid is sucked off, and the adhering salt solution is washed from the crystalline mass by pouring on a layer of ice-cold distilled water, agitating the liquid very gently and then immediately sucking off. This washing may be repeated, but must be carried out with great caution as the crystals are very readily soluble. Recrystallisation may be brought about by dissolving the mass in about an equal volume of distilled water and repeating the freezing and centrifuging as before. The crystals are best removed from the tube while still frozen, and the hæmoglobin may be obtained as a dry powder by keeping this frozen material for a day or two over anhydrous calcium chloride in a vacuum desiccator at $-15°$ C. The ice then sublimes directly into the drying agent, but even at this temperature the hæmoglobin suffers a certain amount of change during the drying process.

The preparation of hæmoglobin without crystallisation. It is urged by those who wish to have hæmoglobin as it exists in the body, that the mere fact of crystallising it is unphysiological, that crystals do not occur in the red blood corpuscle, and that the formation of crystals involves something more far-reaching than mere concentration and something which may not be reversible, that, in fact, hæmoglobin which has been crystallised and redissolved is not the same as the original material. With this point of view I at one time had a good deal of sympathy, and I still think that there is much truth in the general outlook—the chief criticism to which it is open is that there is too much truth in it; for, as we shall see later, it may be doubted whether any hæmoglobin outside the body is governed by quite the same laws as that inside. If it is governed by different laws it will present different properties. Even therefore if the hæmoglobin in a solution be the same as that in the corpuscle, it cannot be assumed that it will act in precisely the same way.

Six or seven years ago, in the endeavour to obtain hæmoglobin solutions, as nearly as possible like those contained in the corpuscle, we naturally tried to make them of great concentration. The observation has often been made that hæmoglobin in the corpuscle was fundamentally different from any obtainable solution because no solution could be made so concentrated as the contents of the corpuscle. That observation is, I think, true of the hæmoglobin of some animals but not of all. Adair has, I believe, obtained hæmoglobin solutions approaching 40 per cent. in concentration.

For practical reasons also it is usually very desirable to have the hæmoglobin in as concentrated a form as possible. Whether for gas measurements or thermal measurements, the greater the concentration of the hæmoglobin the larger the proportion would the readings caused by the effect under consideration bear to those due to adventitious causes and experimental errors.

The solutions used by Barcroft and Roberts had, as stated above, a hæmoglobinometer reading of 70—in other words they were about 9 per cent. hæmoglobin. As time went on and technique improved solutions of considerably greater concentration as well as purity were used. It will be noted that the dialysed solution had been at one period as dilute as 4 per cent. hæmoglobin and had subsequently been concentrated.

More recently an attempt was made in collaboration with Adair [7] to manufacture small quantities of very concentrated hæmoglobin solution, the properties of which—the conductivity, the hydrogen-ion concentration, the dissociation curve and the oxygen capacity—were known, and of these properties more anon. But whilst these experiments had been taking place, another property of the solutions had gradually been forcing itself upon us, namely, their transparency. Some of our solutions were more transparent than others. We therefore subjected them to microscopical examination. We had supposed that in the hæmoglobin solution there might be "shadows" which, owing to the viscosity and the high specific gravity of the solution, it had been impossible to separate by centrifuging. One film which we made rather bore out this view, for when stained with Jenner's stain the solid matter did not take the stain whilst the solution stained red. The nature of the material with which we were working revealed itself in the following way. If a drop of a relatively transparent solution of hæmoglobin be placed on a slide and a coverslip be put on it (thus producing a thin layer of the material) the material presents a very ill-defined appearance. Clearly there is something solid in it, but it is very difficult to say what, or to describe it. If, however, a drop of saline is placed at the side and allowed to diffuse under the coverslip a remarkable transformation takes place. At once the preparation assumes the appearance of blood. The corpuscles are somewhat ill-shapen as is the case when a solution not quite isotonic with it is added to blood, but it is clear that they retain a great part of their hæmoglobin. If, instead of a microscopic preparation, a little of the original dialysed "rather transparent" solution be taken in a test-tube and some salt added, it immediately assumes the appearance of normal blood.

Clearly the solutions with which we had been working were not solutions in the accepted sense at all. They consisted of a mass of corpuscles which as dialysis had proceeded gradually swelled up at the expense of the surrounding fluid till they finally almost lost their refrangibility. Consequently it became possible to see light through the solution as is seen through corpuscles which are pressed together in a hæmatocrit. It now seemed that a possible explanation of the irregular behaviour of our solutions was forthcoming. The dissociation curve of hæmoglobin even within the saltless corpuscle might be essentially different from that of free hæmoglobin in a correspondingly salt-free solution.

The above observations have been expanded by Brown, and indeed a whole literature has grown up around the subject, but it takes us away from the manufacture of hæmoglobin and to the subject of reversible hæmolysis (11), (12).

REFERENCES

(1) FERRY. *Journ. Biol. Chem.* LVII. 819. 1923.

(2) BOHR. *Skand. Arch. f. Physiol.* III. 85. 1892.

(3) BARCROFT AND ROBERTS. *Journ. Physiol.* XXXIX. 143. 1909.

(4) BARCROFT AND HILL. *Journ. Physiol.* XXXIX. 411. 1909–1910.

(5) DUDLEY AND EVANS. *Biochem. Journ.* XV. 487. 1921.

(6) HEIDELBERGER. *Journ. Biol. Chem.* LIII. 31. 1922.

(7) ADAIR, BARCROFT AND BOCK. *Journ. Physiol.* LV. 332. 1921.

(8) VAN SLYKE AND STADIE. *Journ. Biol. Chem.* XLIX. 10. 1921.

(9) STADIE. *Journ. Biol. Chem.* XLI. 237. 1920.

(10) OFFRINGA. *Biochem. Zeitsch.* XXVIII. 106. 1910.

(11) BRINKMAN AND SZENT-GYÖRGYI. *Journ. Physiol.* LVIII. 204. 1923.

(12) BAYLISS, L. E. *Journ. Physiol.* LIX. 47. 1924.

CHAPTER VIII

THE NATURE OF HÆMOGLOBIN SOLUTION

ALGERNON BLACKWOOD(1) gives certain directions as to the way in which an article should be written. You say everything that is worth saying in a line or so at the commencement; you repeat it at somewhat greater length in the next paragraph or two and finally you make a detailed survey of it in the remainder of the article. This injunction at once relieves me of a considerable difficulty for, before going further, it is necessary to make some preliminary statement as to the nature of what is usually called a "hæmoglobin solution," and at the same time it is desirable to defer a final examination of the matter till a later portion of the book.

Here let us suppose that we have a "solution" of hæmoglobin made as indicated in the previous chapter, or even made by simply laking blood, that we have the solution in a closed vessel and that we shake it up with oxygen so as to produce an equilibrium between the hæmoglobin and the oxygen, and let us suppose further that we are about to study the nature of this equilibrium; the question must arise: How many phases are involved? We have in the vessel the gas above the liquid, we have the water, and we have the hæmoglobin. The water cannot be considered as anything but liquid. Does the gas count as a gas? Does the hæmoglobin count as a solid? These questions become the more pertinent because Bayliss(2) has compared the equilibrium between oxygen and hæmoglobin "solutions" with that between carbonic acid gas and solid calcium carbonate.

With regard to the oxygen the matter is simply disposed of. It is only the oxygen which is in solution which counts. The gas above the solution is merely a device for obtaining a given concentration of oxygen in the solution. Once the equilibrium is established the atmosphere above the solution may be removed, as by intercepting a layer of liquid paraffin between the gaseous oxygen and the solution. No change is wrought in the equilibrium, i.e. in the relation between the oxygen chemically combined with the hæmoglobin and that physically dissolved in the water with which the hæmoglobin molecules are in intimate contact.

I have heard the contention that such a treatment of the subject is illegitimate—that the introduction of a layer of paraffin or a glass tap between the hæmoglobin and the oxygen above it produces a fundamental alteration in the system for the following reasons: Suppose (1) you have two vessels, A and B, in which identical solutions of hæmoglobin are exposed to identical atmospheres, the atmosphere and the solution being in each case brought into equilibrium with one another; (2) that in A a layer of material impervious to oxygen is introduced between the gas and the fluid, whilst in B they are left in free contact; and (3) the conditions are altered so that a little oxygen is displaced from the hæmoglobin in each case and goes into the solution. It is contended, and correctly so, that the effect in the two fluids will be different—in A the oxygen will accumulate and produce a greater change of oxygen pressure in•the fluid than before, in B, if the atmosphere is large in volume relatively to that of the hæmoglobin solution, the concentration of oxygen in the solution will remain approximately unchanged. All this is quite true, but if you are discussing an equilibrium, it is beside the mark. Your equilibrium is made and the third supposition above is that, being made, it is then upset. That supposition is irrelevant and the discussion of the subsequent happenings is in the same category as "the flowers that bloom in the spring."

Analogies with what happens when a solid (or liquid in which the gas is insoluble) is exposed to a gas at varying pressures of the latter have no bearing on the present equilibrium—such might be calcium carbonate and CO_2 or mercury and oxygen.

Having eliminated the gaseous phase, the more difficult question arises: Have we a system which consists of a liquid phase composed of water containing oxygen in solution and a solid phase consisting of hæmoglobin; or have we a system which consists of a single liquid phase—the oxygen and the hæmoglobin both being in solution?

The following considerations bear on this point:

(1) If a "solution" be well and truly made, ultra-microscopic examination reveals no foci which disperse the light, apart from such occasional ones as may be due to contamination. It is, I believe, difficult to detect protein aggregates with the ultra-microscope and therefore this test does not carry us very far. Still, if the test had gone the other way, the presence of "solid" bodies would have to be accepted.

(2) All "solutions" of hæmoglobin maintain an osmotic pressure when dialysed in an osmometer permeable to water and salt, but not to hæmoglobin itself.

(3) Such membranes are not easy to prepare because most collodion membranes are to some extent permeable to hæmoglobin. To obtain a satisfactory one it is necessary to make a number and test them—most of them allow more or less of the hæmoglobin to pass through their substance. The hæmoglobin molecules, or some of them, are just about the critical size; if the mesh of the membrane is large they will pass, if small they will not. Nor does a parchment membrane completely retain hæmoglobin. Roberts and I (3), in the manufacture of the solutions of which we shall speak later, and which were made by dialysis in a parchment membrane, found that some of the pigment always escaped and this we could not on every occasion attribute to discrete holes in the parchment. Now that spectroscopic methods have made the use of dilute solutions possible, there would be no difficulty in investigating the equilibrium between oxygen and a solution of hæmoglobin, every molecule of which had traversed a collodion membrane. Indeed, such a study might be well worth while for several reasons, one of which would be the comparison of the hæmoglobin which came through the membrane with that which remained in the membrane. It raises the question whether in a hæmoglobin solution all the molecules are of the same size, or whether they are of all sorts of sizes. It is clear that in the literature there are two quite different conceptions of what a hæmoglobin solution is like. The one is that each molecule is similar to its fellow as one supposes to be the case with simple substances, the other is that the molecules are of all sorts of magnitudes, the smallest containing one atom of iron and having a molecular weight in the neighbourhood of 17,000.

The largest such molecules may attain a size to which the term "solid" is applicable. This view of hæmoglobin as existing in the form of aggregates of all sorts of sizes, but with an average size of somewhere between two and three times the possible minimum, was first put forward as a working hypothesis by A. V. Hill (4) and will have to be referred to later in another and a very important connection. Meanwhile it suggests to the reader a view which has become rather fashionable of recent years, namely, that there is no fundamental distinction between a true solution, a colloidal solution, and a suspension, the one state of matter passing imperceptibly into the other. Such a view may be quite correct if held on a basis of understanding, but of course it would be intolerable to use a fashionable idea for the purpose of cloaking our ignorance as to the exact state of the system with which we are dealing.

Let us take a single instance of the sort of difficulty which lies before us. Suppose we consider the equilibrium of oxygen, hæmoglobin and oxyhæmoglobin, all in *solution* in water, and supposing the hæmoglobin and oxyhæmoglobin are present as single molecules, the simple reaction

$$Hb + O_2 \rightleftarrows HbO_2$$

is represented mathematically by a rectangular hyperbola—a fact which is shown in detail in Chapter x. If, on the other hand, the hæmoglobin and oxyhæmoglobin are conceived of as solids and in a different phase from the oxygen, the law of mass action would indicate that there should be a critical pressure of oxygen below which all the hæmoglobin would be reduced and above which it would all be oxidised. That at least is what might be expected if a sufficiently fine powder of crystalline hæmoglobin were exposed to gaseous oxygen. Now, if we are going to study the equilibrium of these substances, which formula are we to adopt as being correct? The dissociation curve cannot be both a continuous and a discontinuous ascent. If the passage from a simple unimolecular solution to a solid is a gradual one with no fundamental break in it, there should be a corresponding gradual transition from the hyperbola to the discontinuous curve. It may be so. At all events it may be worth considering the matter if a certain assumption is made, namely, that should molecules unite to form an aggregate that particular aggregate is either completely oxidised or completely reduced. Under such circumstances the reaction is represented by the formula

$$\frac{y}{100} = \frac{Kx^n}{1 + Kx^n},$$

where y is the percentage of the hæmoglobin which is oxidised, x is the oxygen pressure, K is the equilibrium constant of the reaction, and n is the average number of molecules, each capable of uniting with two atoms of oxygen, which form an aggregate. If $n = 1$, the curve obtained from the above reaction is a hyperbola, if n is greater than 1, the curve becomes inflected and increasingly so with an increase in the value of n. In Fig. 14 a number of curves are drawn with different values for n, it being assumed in each case that at 10 mm. pressure of oxygen the hæmoglobin is 50 per cent. saturated. In the limiting case the inflection would be so great as to make the curve vertical for most of its length, that is to say 10 mm. would be a critical pressure at above which all the hæmoglobin would be oxy-hæmoglobin and below which it would be reduced hæmoglobin.

In the case of hæmoglobin it is particularly desirable to have clear views as to whether it really is in solution or not, because the whole modern theory of hæmoglobin which contemplates the substance as one which presents the properties of an acid and a base in varying degrees under different circumstances, assumes fundamentally that the substance is in solution, otherwise it would not dissociate into hydrogen, hydroxyl and hæmoglobin ions.

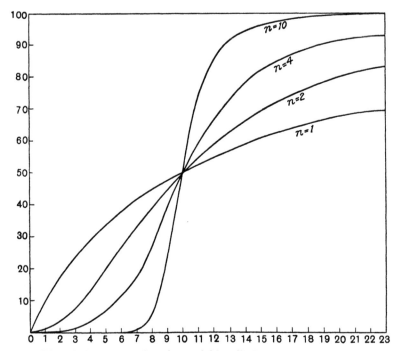

FIG. 14. Dissociation curves of oxyhæmoglobin, all 50 per cent. saturated at 10 mm. pressure, but with varying values of n.

Another criterion which is sometimes cited of whether a substance is or is not in solution is its power to exert an osmotic pressure. What justification had we a while back for stating that hæmoglobin possessed this property? The answer cannot be given without going in some detail into a rather chequered chapter of physiological research. The importance of the issues involved was recognised by

Hüfner (5), and the question like some others was "settled" by him. His observations, made in collaboration with Gansser, showed that a so-called solution of hæmoglobin exerted an osmotic pressure which corresponded to a molecular weight for the substance of about 17,000. This highly satisfactory result left no doubt in the minds of the authors that hæmoglobin existed in true solution and that the molecule was the simplest possible, i.e. one which contained a single atom of iron. On this basis a 1 per cent. solution of hæmoglobin would have an osmotic pressure of about 10 mm. of mercury, which was about what Hüfner and Gansser found it to be.

Reid (6) previously had made similar measurements. Exactly why his results were called in question by Hüfner I have never quite known. Of course they appeared somewhat anomalous but they showed a healthy scepticism—a scepticism which in Reid I have always admired since I heard the following story about him—which story may of course be apocryphal. Reid read a research which had to do with diffusion or vitalism or something of the kind. Armed with a soda-water bottle and two frogs Reid pursued the writer round the European capital in which his laboratory was situated in order that the author of the work might have the opportunity of demonstrating the phenomenon which he had described, but as I heard it the author always had a train to catch or some equally urgent call afoot. That, however, is a digression, I only wish to indicate that such a combination of enthusiasm and energy cannot in the long run go unrewarded. Certainly in the matter of hæmoglobin's osmotic properties Waymouth Reid entirely got the better of Hüfner. As the result of a most careful piece of work which is less quoted than it should be, Reid concluded that the osmotic pressure of hæmoglobin was but a third of what Hüfner and Gansser made it out to be. Reid obtained very uniform and consistent results.

It is just at this point of consistency that the problem took the next turn, for Roaf (7), who worked at the subject in Liverpool, made an important advance in pointing out that the osmotic pressure of hæmoglobin could not be regarded as a constant quantity, but that it varied with the nature of the solvent of the hæmoglobin, whether for instance it was acid, alkaline, etc. Among Roaf's results was the apparent anomaly that the osmotic pressure settled down on occasions to something which corresponded to less than one molecular weight.

Roaf, I remember, very kindly showed me his osmometers and

quite convinced me that these apparently anomalous results were the opening of a new chapter with regard to the osmotic pressure of hæmoglobin.

It need hardly be said that the problem bristles with difficulties. Had it not done so I doubt if it would have thrown its spell over Adair[8], [9], who has carried out the most recent and the most complete work in this field. Perhaps before discussing Adair's work a word or two might be said about these difficulties. They fall into several categories, the first of which is that of the actual measurements. These measurements are two, that of the concentration of the solution and that of the height to which it rises in the osmometer. It is not easy to measure the concentration of a hæmoglobin solution. Reid, and later, Hüfner, used the spectrophotometer for this purpose; their method is now probably of historical interest and may be found in a chapter by Gamgee in Schafer's[10] text-book. Stoddard and Adair[11] applied a method based on measurements of the refractive index. This method had previously been used to measure the concentrations of other proteins. It was duly checked by chemical analysis.

The question may, however, be asked: Why not take the oxygen capacity as a measure of the concentration of hæmoglobin? A trifling doubt in the quantity of oxygen which unites with each gram of hæmoglobin is not very material if the point at issue is whether the osmotic pressure is in the end going to correspond to Hb or Hb_4. There are some other considerations, however. Account must be taken of that ill-understood form of hæmoglobin which does not part with its oxygen either in the ferricyanide or in the Van Slyke apparatus. Moreover, reliable oxygen readings can only be obtained from hæmoglobin solutions of considerable concentration; a part of the merit of Adair's work is that it deals with dilute, as well as strong solutions. The difficulty of measuring the concentration, then, is the first which has to be overcome in the estimation of the osmotic pressure of hæmoglobin. As in all such matters the position cannot really be regarded as satisfactory until two independent methods give results which agree. Till then we must take our choice and as between the spectrophotometer and the refractometer, the latter would seem to be the more desirable.

Now let us pass to the second difficulty of actual measurement— that of obtaining a reliable reading for the pressure itself. Here one is on the horns of a dilemma. If you do not keep your solutions long enough in the osmometer an equilibrium will never be established and the final osmotic pressure will never be obtained. If, on the other hand, you take sufficient time for the attainment of a final equilibrium your solution may "go bad" and you may have quite a different number of molecules from that with which you started.

One way of meeting such difficulties—evidently not very satisfactory—is frankly to give up the idea of obtaining equilibrium, to set a time limit to the experiment, to take a series of readings of the osmotic pressure at suitable intervals, and to trust to extrapolation for the final result. Something, again, can be done to accelerate the attainment of a final pressure in the osmometer by resort to the expedient of prophecy. An initial pressure, adjudged about equal to what the ultimate pressure will be, is established artificially by making the osmometer work against a mercury column. This process is not satisfactory either, because after all it does not hasten the processes which are going to make for finality.

Naturally the larger the surface relative to the volume of fluid in the osmometer, the more rapidly will finality be reached, and of course the more completely the fluids are stirred the better. When I think of the dialyser which I used in order to obtain salt-free hæmoglobin (3)—a parchment sausage about 2 feet long and perhaps 3 or 4 inches in circumference placed in a jar containing half a score of litres of distilled water, and agitated by being pulled up and down by an engine—and when I compare that apparatus with the beautifully simple and efficient osmometers of Adair (8), with collodion membranes of texture so exquisite as just, and only just, to retain the hæmoglobin molecule, yet capable of standing high pressures, membranes possessing a sufficient relative surface to allow of the maximum rate of dialysis, then I realise how far Adair has gone—I appreciate a little of what lies behind the apparently naïve statement in one of his papers: "After a few years' practice the proportion of failures was less than 10 per cent." (8) A few years' practice! And it was not that the first membrane which Adair made was a bad one. I saw him make it. A biochemist, for whom I have a great respect, came to our laboratory; he had had much experience as a manufacturer of membranes but he was making "heavy weather" of it; his wife, for whom I also have a great respect, came along and "went one better." Adair watched them both: at long last and in silence he took some of the collodion, set a rod spinning, poured on the fluid, and lo! a membrane of no mean order.

A few lines back I referred to the precision with which Adair controls the texture of his membranes. I should like to elaborate this point and, if I could, help the reader to the attainment of a like skill; but I doubt whether such knowledge is susceptible of communication through the channel of the "written word." The alternative to acquiring it by a few *years* of practice, without Adair, is a few *months* of practice with him, and here we have at once the justification and the condemnation of research schools. Before the days of printing scholars went from university to university to learn by personal contact what the great teachers had to teach; the distribution of knowledge by the vehicle of printed books has reduced the necessity of personal contact to a minimum. In science, however, there is to be considered not merely what the teacher can say in his lecture—which can be printed—but the way he works with his own two hands or, if you like, the expression of his personality in his technique: that can only be acquired by observation. That is largely the justification of a research school, but once the school becomes so large that the teacher ceases himself to work, the school must surely be living to a large extent on its past. I will not put it more strongly than this: when the head of a school finds himself so engrossed in organising the researches of his pupils as to do none himself it is worth his while to take an occasional glance at the wall to see whether, from under the whitewash, he cannot discern the words commencing to appear, "Mene, mene, tekel, Eupharsin."

It was, I think, "the Quaker" in Adair which enabled him to overcome the technical difficulties of a problem which had proved too difficult for many a previous worker. The desire for finality and truth excluded such processes as extrapolation, whilst aversion to "creaturely activity[1]" demanded that to the process of osmosis should be accorded as much time as was necessary for its completion. The solution of the problem—as a technical one—lay in carrying out the whole experiment in cold storage. Where others at room temperature thought and worked in terms of days, Adair was prepared to take months at 0° C. He was fortunate in having the facilities of the Cambridge Low Temperature Station for his purpose. In it time is no particular object, the hæmoglobin neither becomes infected nor deteriorates and an ultimate equilibrium can be obtained.

---

[1] A term used by the early Quakers to signify the use of artificial pressure in order to accelerate the natural process of spiritual development.

So much for the technical difficulties, great enough, but less than those imposed by the nature of hæmoglobin itself.

What if hæmoglobin has no osmotic pressure, the pressure which is set up being due to adherent salts? In such an event hæmoglobin would not be in solution; but in such a case also the particular conditions which Adair demanded (8) would probably not have been complied with. They were (1) that successive samples of hæmoglobin should give the same value under similar conditions; (2) that if, when final equilibrium had been reached, the pressure were disturbed in either direction, it should return to the previous value; and (3) that the pressure should be maintained at a constant level for a considerable time. Hæmoglobin gave results which fell so well within the set limitations, as to leave no doubt that it did of itself exert a definite osmotic pressure.

Definite! Yes, but the osmotic pressure was a function of the conditions under which it was measured, as indeed Roaf has discovered. How could this be? The idea which underlay Hüfner's work and, as I suppose, Waymouth Reid's, was that the hæmoglobin molecule was just a molecule—as it might be urea or sugar but vastly larger. How much larger, was what they set themselves to discover. The modern view is different, it is that hæmoglobin is something which in alkaline solutions behaves like an acid uniting with a base and in acid solutions behaves like an alkali, uniting with an acid. Picture it then in a dilute solution of sodium hydrate, forming a salt—sodium hæmoglobinate; the precise number of gram atomic weights of sodium with which each 17,000 gram units of hæmoglobin unites need not be discussed here, but it may be quite considerable, say ten, if the solution is sufficiently alkaline. A true salt is formed, that is to say the sodium atoms are at least partially in the ionised condition as also is the hæmoglobin. The osmotic pressure of course will depend upon the number of ions. Within limits the more alkaline the solution the greater will be the osmotic pressure of the sodium hæmoglobinate. Hence in an alkaline solution the osmotic pressure will fall as the alkalinity diminishes. The same is true of an acid solution where the hæmoglobin acts as a base and attaches to itself numerous acid ions, the less the concentration of hydrogen ions the less the osmotic pressure caused by the hæmoglobin. At the isoelectric point therefore of the hæmoglobin (about pH 6·8) the hæmoglobin should on this theory exert its minimum osmotic pressure (9). It is not very easy to obtain hæmoglobin quite free from base and at the same time untouched by acid, for it very easily deteriorates in acid solution. The object is best attained by treating the hæmoglobin with carbonic acid, which, if bubbled long enough, seizes all the sodium for the formation of sodium carbonate; this, as it appears, dialyses away. Having freed the hæmoglobin from sodium it is then possible to dialyse it against distilled water, thus avoiding questions of the unequal distribution of salts on either side of the membrane. This operation is one of the greatest delicacy, as will be gleaned from the following statement: "In one experiment traces of carbon dioxide in the air, due to the respiration of a small sample of fruit and vegetables placed in the same cold store, doubled the osmometer readings within twenty-four hours [8]."

The uniformity of Adair's results is remarkable considering the difficulties against which he was working.

The following table shows a series of experiments:

Osmotic pressure per 1 % Hb	Concentration of Hb per cent.	Species
2·5	1·7	Man
3·2	4·0	,,
3·0	1·2	,,
3·0	1·3	,,
3·0	6·8	,,
2·9	2·7	Horse
3·1	1·3	,,
3·1	2·4	,,
2·9	4·8	Ox
2·8	2·2	Sheep (laked)
2·9	3·8	,, (cryst. with ether)
2·8	2·8	,, (crystallised)

In discussing Hüfner's results we said that a solution in which each molecule had a weight of 17,000 grams would in theory yield an osmotic pressure of 10 mm. for every per cent. of hæmoglobin. Adair's result is something quite different from that. It is lower even than Waymouth Reid's and corresponds to a molecular weight of approximately 67,000, i.e. to a molecule of Hb_4 [9].

The fact that a dilute and strictly neutral hæmoglobin solution consists of molecules with an average molecular weight of somewhere in the region of 70,000 seems to be one of the fundamental facts on which any theory of the nature of hæmoglobin must be based.

Having once attained that fixed point one may ask: What if the solution is not dilute, and is not strictly neutral? What if it contains salts? These three factors, salts, hydrogen-ion concentration and hæmoglobin concentration, have effects on the osmotic pressure which are so interwoven that it is not possible to consider each one quite separately from the other two. Nevertheless we may first say something about the effect of salts. Salts have a wonderful effect in stabilising the osmotic pressure. Any dilute solution of hæmoglobin which contains more than the merest trace of salts (about ·01 molecular), of whatever hydrogen-ion concentration, has an osmotic pressure of about 2·6 mm. Hg for each per cent.[1] of hæmoglobin present. When one gets to solutions so free from salts as to have a less saline content than ·01 molecular the osmotic pressure rapidly rises (12).

It follows therefore that if the effect of varying the hydrogen-ion concentration is to be brought about the solution must be salt free. Fig. 17 shows that in a salt-free solution the osmotic pressure is 2·6 for each per cent. of hæmoglobin at the isoelectric point, but that on either side of neutrality the pressure rises rapidly—on the alkaline side owing to the formation of sodium hæmoglobinate, on the acid side owing to the formation of hæmoglobin chloride (9).

The above statements apply to solutions of less hæmoglobin concentration than about 4 per cent. Above this strength the osmotic pressure for each per cent. of hæmoglobin rises. At concentrations such as are found in the red blood corpuscle, 30–40 per cent., the osmotic pressure is much higher relatively, being about 5 mm. or even more for each per cent. (12)

REFERENCES

(1) ALGERNON BLACKWOOD. *Episodes before Thirty*. London, 1923.
(2) BAYLISS. *Principles of General Physiology*, XXI. 615. 1924.
(3) BARCROFT AND ROBERTS. *Journ. Physiol.* XXXIX. 143. 1909.
(4) HILL, A. V. *Journ. Physiol.* XL. iv (Proceedings). 1910.
—— *Biochem. Journ.* VII. 471. 1913.
(5) HÜFNER AND GANSSER. *Arch. f. Anat. u. Physiol.* p. 209. 1907.
(6) REID. *Journ. Physiol.* XXXIII. 12. 1905.
(7) ROAF. *Journ. Physiol.* XXXVIII. i (Proceedings). 1909.
(8) ADAIR. *Proc. Roy. Soc.* A. CVIII. 627. 1925.
(9) ADAIR. *Proc. Roy. Soc.* A. CIX. 292. 1925.
(10) SCHAFER. *Text Book of Physiology*, I. 234. 1898.
(11) STODDARD AND ADAIR. *Journ. Biol. Chem.* LVII. 437. 1923.
(12) BARCROFT. *Journ. Chem. Soc.* p. 1146. May, 1926.

[1] The strength of the solution may be measured without drying the hæmoglobin either spectrophotometrically (10) or refractometrically (11).

CHAPTER IX

THE MOLECULAR WEIGHT OF HÆMOGLOBIN

FROM the chemist's point of view the molecular weight of hæmoglobin is one of those things which is of first importance. Yet it has proved most illusive. Needless to say almost every worker has been anxious to determine it, but the determination has till recently proved a veritable will-o'-the-wisp and even now the subject is surrounded with many difficulties. The thermal method at one time held out great hopes. The perusal of Chapters XVI and XVII shows to how small an extent these hopes have been realised. There is no question of vapour pressure. We turn therefore to the osmotic pressure. We know as a starting-point that the least possible molecular weight—that which contains 56 grams of iron—would be somewhere around 16,700. If then we call the molecular weight $(16,700)_n$, what is the value of n?

I may pass rather rapidly over the work of Hüfner and Gansser[1], who came to the conclusion that the osmotic pressure of a 1 per cent. solution of hæmoglobin would be 10 mm. of mercury—a result which would give a value of $n = 1$. By what happy accident Hüfner and Gansser arrived at this result is likely to remain a mystery. Waymouth Reid[2], in a research which is too little quoted, concluded that 3 was the nearest whole number to his determinations of n. Roaf[3] made the material but rather depressing discovery that n might appear to be almost anything—less than unity, for instance—according to the circumstances in which the measurements were made. It has remained for Adair[4] to reduce to some sort of order the apparently chaotic readings which were found. The possibilities of adsorbed salts, of variable ionisation of the hydrogen or sodium ions, of membrane potentials, of polymerisation of the hæmoglobin, of the onset of putrefaction, of the attainment of a true equilibrium, etc., all had to be taken into account. Take the last two considerations, the avoidance of putrefactive changes and the attainment of equilibrium. In ordinary circumstances it proved quite impossible to complete a measurement in a time so short as to guarantee freedom from putrefaction. This difficulty was overcome by working at $-0.6°C.$, at which temperature a hæmoglobin solution remains good indefinitely.

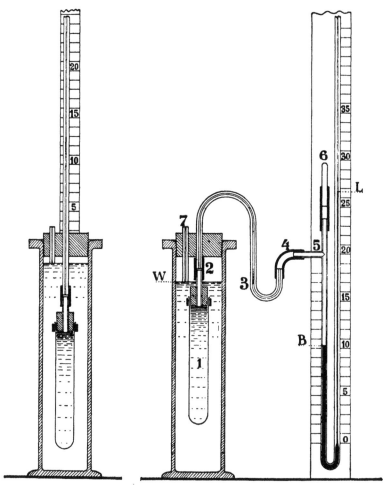

Fig. 15. Osmometer, Type D (left), with straight column of solution for measuring
pressure. Scale in centimetres. Osmometer, Type C (right), for high pressures
with mercury manometer: (1) A rigid collodion tube, 20 c.c. capacity, in jar
holding 500 c.c. of outer liquid. (2) Rubber connection. The glass tube from
(2) to (3) is filled with liquid paraffin. Beyond (3) there is water. (4) Rubber
connection with clip (not shown here). (5) Glass T-tube, with water down to
level B. (6) Glass rod in rubber tube, for adjusting the pressure. (7) Glass tube,
open to air, or fitted with a soda-lime tube. W = level of outer liquid; B = leve
of mercury in manometer limb, 6 mm. in diameter; L = level of mercury in
manometer limb, 0·7 mm. in diameter. Above the mercury at L there is a dro
of lactic acid.

The time factor looms almost as large in Adair's determinations as in those of Hartridge and Roughton. The latter measure events which take place in a fraction of 1/1000 of a second; Adair's osmometric determinations each require a fraction of a year. The work is being carried on in the Low Temperature Station at Cambridge, where Sir Wm. Hardy kindly allows Adair to set up his osmometers. Such work must be very slow, but already enough information has been obtained to be of considerable interest. Adair will show you a model in which the osmotic pressure in a 1 per cent. solution of hæmoglobin is represented vertically whilst the hydrogen-ion concentration and the saline concentration of the solvent are as the horizontal co-ordinates. Over a great area of this model the osmotic pressure

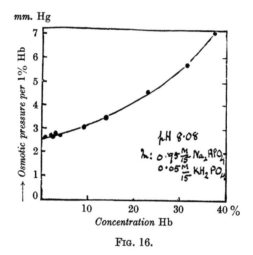

FIG. 16.

of the hæmoglobin works out uniformly at 2·6 mm. of mercury, even though the pH and the salt concentration vary [5], [6]. This figure is given if the solution is not more than 4 per cent. hæmoglobin or is not of less saline concentration than 0·01 molecular. Where a different and higher osmotic pressure than 2·6 mm. is given per 1 per cent. of hæmoglobin, as in cases where the concentration of Hb is more than 4 per cent. (Fig. 16) or the pigment is dissolved in salt solution of greater dilution than 0·01 M (Fig. 17), Adair finds a cause which satisfies him. If we accept his estimate, the value of n would be 4 and the molecular weight of hæmoglobin about 68,000.

Turning from the osmotic pressure, another indirect method of measuring the molecular weight would be by depression of the freezing-point. If Adair's calculation may be relied upon the depression of the freezing-point would be of the order of 0·00001° C., a quantity so small as to put the measurement outside the realm of profitable research.

But if the recognised methods for the indirect determination of molecular weights have, with the exception of osmometry, failed, there is some compensation in the knowledge that an entirely new and very beautiful method has been born of the desire to know the molecular weight of hæmoglobin. Certainly chemistry owes much

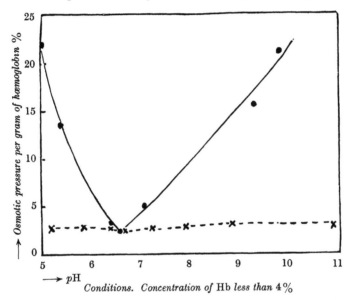

Conditions.   Concentration of Hb less than 4%

FIG. 17.   • = distilled water.   × = solution of saline concentration greater than 0·01 M.

to hæmoglobin in that this substance only yields up its secrets to those who arm themselves with novel and beautiful methods of investigation. None could be more fascinating than the method of determination of molecular weight by ultracentrifugalisation. This technique is due to Professor Svedberg[8] of Upsala. I am told that the information was won at a cost of "thousands of pounds" and I can well believe it.

The reader will be nearer to an understanding of Svedberg's work if he considers the conditions prevailing in the atmosphere. Close to the earth the air is densest, as an ascent is made the air becomes increasingly more rare. These facts do not change with time. An equilibrium is therefore maintained between two forces acting on the gases of the atmosphere, one force is that of gravity, which attracts the air to the centre of the earth, the other is that of diffusion, which tends to dissipate the air uniformly over the universe. Now the mathematical expression of the velocity of diffusion contains the molecular weight of the gas, that of the influence of gravity on it does not. An equilibrium between the two may therefore be represented by an equation in which the molecular weight appears on one side, and one side only; therefore if all the other quantities in the equation are known, the molecular weight of the gas may be calculated. Nor was Svedberg's the first important application of this principle. By invoking its aid Perrin performed his classical research on the sedimentation of gamboge particles into layers of increasing density from an originally uniform solution.

Hæmoglobin molecules will not sediment, some force much more powerful than gravity being required to divert their path in a uniform direction. At very high speeds of rotation, however, centrifugal force was made by Svedberg to effect this object.

The theory then put simply is as follows: If a solution of hæmoglobin is centrifuged with sufficient rapidity it will cease to be homogeneous and the molecules of hæmoglobin will separate out as particles would do in an ordinary solution. Normally the solution is kept homogeneous because the forces of diffusion overpower all others, and the rate at which the hæmoglobin separates when centrifuged depends upon the degree to which centrifugal force can overcome diffusion. Now, of these two forces which can be brought into equilibrium, one, the rate of sedimentation of the hæmoglobin, does not depend upon the molecular weight, the other, the rate of diffusion, does. Therefore balancing the one against the other we get an equation which contains the molecular weight on the one side and not on the other. Clearly if we can measure all the other things in the equation we can calculate the molecular weight[1]. Fortunately such things as do not cancel out can be measured. They are:

(1) The concentrations (c_1 and c_2) of the solution at two points, these points being at known distances (x_1 and x_2) from the centre of rotation.

(2) The absolute temperature (T).

(3) The speed of the centrifuge, giving the angular velocity (ω).

[1] The formula for finding the molecular weight M is
$$M = \frac{2RT \left(\log_e c_1/c_2\right)}{\omega^2 \left(1 - V\rho\right)\left(x_1 - x_2\right)\left(x_1 + x_2\right)}.$$

(4) The partial specific volume of the solute (V).

(5) The density of the solvent (ρ).

The rate of centrifugalisation is in the region of 10,000 revolutions per minute, which is responsible for a force of about 6000 times that of gravity. The critical measurement is of course that of the concentration of the hæmoglobin at different portions of the tube. In order to understand how this is carried out the reader must first appreciate the nature of the tube and of the centrifuge. The centrifuge consists of a whirling disc of ebonite. In this disc are cut eight circular holes. Fig. 18 shows the arrangement. Four of the holes in the disc

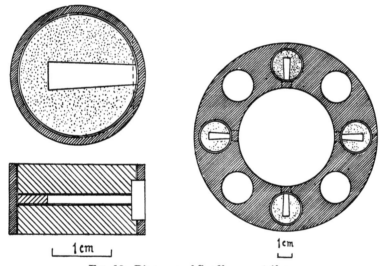

1 cm

1 cm

Fig. 18. Diagrams of Svedberg centrifuge.

contain what I have so far called "tubes," but what should be called cells because they present flat surfaces when looked at from above and from below. The actual cavity in each cell which holds the hæmoglobin solution is only a little over 1 cm. in length. The whole is arranged so that the disc and its contents, with the exception of the hæmoglobin solution, is opaque, and thus a camera placed above the cell will photograph the extent to which the solution has sedimented.

The photographs are taken while the disc is rotating. The experiment lasts six hours. Experiments of this character have been carried out on carboxyhæmoglobin and on methæmoglobin in dilute solutions.

The results may be expressed in terms of the value of n, the calculated number by which 16,700 must be multiplied to give the true molecular weight.

Value of n

Number of experiments ...	COHb		Met-Hb	
	Series I	Series II	Series I	Series II
	9	10	8	12
Maximum ...	4·59	4·58	4·56	4·07
Minimum ...	3·49	3·98	3·79	3·19
Mean	4·06	4·25	4·18	3·73

Considering the amazing boldness of the technique it will be agreed that these experiments leave no doubt that in the strength of solution used the value of n is 4. The results of Adair and Svedberg are therefore in exact agreement.

There is one more thing to be said: a given value of n might merely be the average of a widely distributed range of values of n for different aggregates. Adair's results rendered this improbable. According to Svedberg's, there was no suggestion of differential ultracentrifugalisation in his tubes. Svedberg and Nichols report that they have also confirmed Adair's determination which showed that n was constant over a considerable range of hydrogen-ion concentration[9].

REFERENCES

(1) Hüfner and Gansser. *Arch. f. Anat. u. Physiol.* p. 209. 1907.
(2) Reid. *Journ. Physiol.* xxxiii. 12. 1905.
(3) Roaf. *Journ. Physiol.* xxxviii. i (Proceedings). 1909.
—— *Quart. Journ. Exper. Physiol.* iii. 75. 1910.
(4) Adair. *Proc. Roy. Soc.* A. cviii. 627. 1925.
(5) Adair. *Proc. Roy. Soc.* A. cix. 292. 1925.
(6) Adair. *Proc. Camb. Phil. Soc. Biol.* i. 75. 1924.
(7) Adair quoted by Barcroft. *Journ. Chem. Soc.* p. 1146. May, 1926.
[For other Adair references, see Chap. i.]
(8) Svedberg. *Journ. Amer. Chem. Soc.* xlviii. 430. 1926.
[For other Svedberg references, see Chap. i.]
(9) Svedberg and Nichols. *Journ. Amer. Chem. Soc.* xlix. 2920. 1927.

CHAPTER X

THE DISSOCIATION CURVE OF HÆMOGLOBIN

If a hæmoglobin solution be shaken up with oxygen the hæmoglobin unites with a definite quantity of the gas, which is in the proportion of 32 grams of oxygen to each 56 grams of iron in the hæmoglobin. However much stress we may lay upon this fact—and we cannot lay too much stress upon it—the most elementary consideration of the hæmoglobin in the circulation reveals the fact that it is always united with less oxygen than the total amount possible.

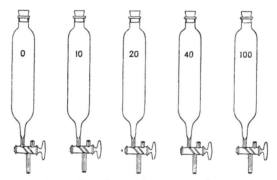

Fig. 19. The numbers denote the pressure of oxygen in mm.

The next step therefore, if we are to regard oxyhæmoglobin as a chemical compound, is to enquire whether we can reconcile the fact that hæmoglobin in the body unites, now with more, now with less oxygen, with the known laws of chemical action.

The most obvious law which might illuminate this problem is the law of mass action. Our enquiry therefore resolves itself into this: granted a solution which contains (1) oxygen, (2) oxyhæmoglobin, and (3) reduced hæmoglobin, does the amount of oxyhæmoglobin depend upon the concentration of oxygen in the solution? The answer to this question can only be supplied by experiment. The experiment is not a difficult one. It is easy to obtain solutions of hæmoglobin containing known quantities of oxygen in solution, for the concentration of oxygen in the solution depends directly upon the oxygen pressure of the atmosphere with which the solution is in equilibrium. If α be the volume of oxygen which is dissolved in

1 c.c. of the solution at the temperature of the experiment and at 760 mm. pressure, the concentration of oxygen at any other pressure p is $p \dfrac{\alpha}{760}$. The experiment, then, will consist in exposing portions of hæmoglobin solution to various atmospheres containing known pressures of oxygen and subsequently determining the amounts of oxy- and reduced hæmoglobin in each sample after an equilibrium has been established between the hæmoglobin and the atmosphere. Suppose we have five closed vessels each containing a small quantity of hæmoglobin solution and also at the same time oxygen at the following pressures, namely 0, 10, 20, 40 and 100 mm. of mercury (Fig. 19). After the fluids had been shaken up thoroughly at 38° C. the concentrations of oxygen would be

(1)	(2)	(3)	(4)	(5)
$0 \times \dfrac{\alpha}{760}$	$10 \dfrac{\alpha}{760}$	$20 \dfrac{\alpha}{760}$	$40 \dfrac{\alpha}{760}$	$100 \dfrac{\alpha}{760}$ c.c.

That is:

$$0 \qquad \cdot00029 \qquad \cdot00058 \qquad \cdot00116 \qquad \cdot0029 \text{ c.c.}$$

of oxygen in each c.c. of fluid.

Now we must find out what proportion of the hæmoglobin is oxyhæmoglobin, and the following are figures such as we should obtain:

Vessel	(1)	(2)	(3)	(4)	(5)
	0 %	55 %	72 %	84 %	92 %

The best idea we can get of the relation of these numbers to one another is to place the following picture before our eyes. Supposing the hæmoglobin in each case to be in a cylindrical tube and that the oxy- and reduced hæmoglobin could be separated from one another, the former being red and sinking to the bottom and the latter purple and rising to the top, we should obtain five cylinders as shown in Fig. 20 corresponding to the oxygen pressures in the five tonometers.

We are impelled to ask whether any definite relationship exists between these quantities of oxyhæmoglobin and the oxygen pressures to which they correspond. In doing so we must bear in mind that we shall shortly be face to face with a very serious position, for the very relationship which we are about to investigate is defined by the law of mass action itself, and should the relation as found not agree with that as prescribed, our theory must be abandoned and some other explanation of the properties of hæmoglobin must be

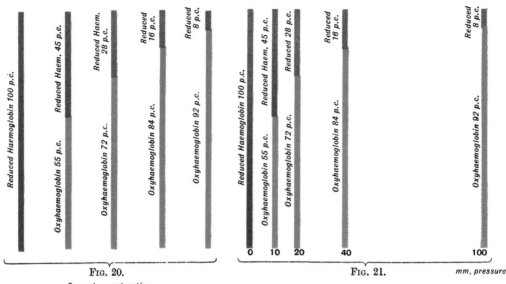

Fig. 20.   Fig. 21.   *mm. pressure*

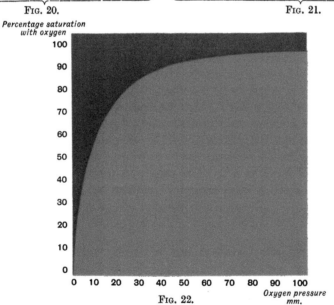

Fig. 22.

Fig. 20.—Percentage saturation of haemoglobin with oxygen at 37° C. corresponding to oxygen pressures of 0, 10, 20, 40 and 100 mm. of oxygen respectively.

Fig. 21.—The same spaced with the oxygen pressure as the abscissa.

Fig. 22.—Dissociation curve representing the equilibrium between oxygen, oxyhaemoglobin (red) and reduced haemoglobin (purple).

found. Let us introduce the element of pressure quantitatively by spacing the cylinders apart from one another at distances which are proportional to the concentrations (or pressure) of oxygen dissolved in the solution, as is done in Fig. 21.

By joining the points which divide the blue and red portions of the cylinders we obtain a curve which relates the percentage of oxyhæmoglobin to the concentration of oxygen dissolved in the fluid at all concentrations of oxygen between 0 and ·0029 c.c., and consequently to all pressures of oxygen between 0 and 100 mm. This curve representing the equilibrium between oxygen and hæmoglobin is called the dissociation curve of oxyhæmoglobin. It is shown in Fig. 22.

Let us now turn from the observed properties of hæmoglobin to the other side of the question, namely the requirements of the law of mass action. This law has been stated quantitatively by Guldberg and Waage in the following terms: "The velocity of chemical change is proportional to the product of the active masses of the reacting substances." The chemical change is conceived as taking place in both directions at the same time, that is to say oxyhæmoglobin is all the time being formed and being broken up, and we therefore have two changes taking place at one and the same time, (1) the formation, (2) the breakdown of oxyhæmoglobin. Since these changes balance one another, the whole system being in equilibrium, the velocities of the two changes are equal. Taking first the formation of oxyhæmoglobin: the reacting substances are reduced hæmoglobin and oxygen and the velocity of their reaction is proportional, says the law, to the *product* of their concentrations in the solution. If C_O be the concentration of oxygen and C_R of reduced hæmoglobin, then the velocity of the reaction is proportional to, or is equal to, a constant k multiplied by the product of C_R and C_O

$$= k\,(C_R \times C_O).$$

As regards the other phase of the reaction—the breakdown of oxyhæmoglobin—there is but one active substance, namely oxy-hæmoglobin; let its concentration be C_H, then the velocity of the reaction is k', another constant, multiplied by C_H. Taking the two together, we have

$$k\,(C_R \times C_O) = k'C_H.$$

The concentration of oxygen as we have already stated is $p \times \dfrac{a}{760}$, where p is the oxygen pressure to which the solution is subjected and α the coefficient of solubility, therefore

$$\frac{k}{k'} \times \frac{\alpha}{760} \times p \times C_R = C_H,$$

and replacing all the constants by one constant K,

$$K.p.C_R = C_H.$$

If the concentrations of oxy- and reduced hæmoglobin are regarded as percentages of the total concentration of hæmoglobin, then

$$C_H = 100 - C_R,$$
$$K.p.C_R = 100 - C_R,$$
$$p.C_R + \frac{C_R}{K} = \frac{100}{K},$$
$$\left(p + \frac{1}{K}\right) C_R = \frac{100}{K}.$$

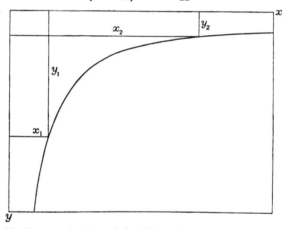

Fig. 23. Rectangular hyperbola. The products of x and y, such as x_1y_1, x_2y_2, for all points are equal.

If we write y for C_R and x for $\left(p + \frac{1}{K}\right)$, we obtain the relationship $xy = $ a constant, namely $\frac{100}{K}$. If we now construct a curve plotting y vertically and x horizontally, and observing the condition that for any point the product of x and y must be constant, we obtain a curve known as a rectangular hyperbola.

This curve does not at first sight relate the concentration of reduced hæmoglobin (C_R) to the pressure p, but to something else, namely $p + \dfrac{1}{K}$. It remains for us to find out what the relation of C_R to p is.

Consider the special case in which $C_R = 100$, i.e. all the hæmoglobin is reduced hæmoglobin,

$$\left(p + \frac{1}{K}\right) C_R = \frac{100}{K},$$

$$\left(p + \frac{1}{K}\right) 100 = \frac{100}{K},$$

$$\therefore p = 0.$$

The distance AB (Fig. 24) in that case $= \dfrac{1}{K}$. Hence the distance from BB' of any point on the hyperbola is a measure of the pressure.

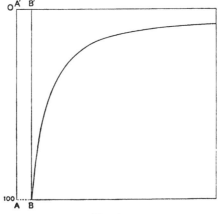

FIG. 24.

We have therefore derived the following information from the law of mass action. If the reaction is a chemical one involving single molecules only, the relation of the oxygen pressure to the percentage of oxy- to total hæmoglobin is capable of being represented as a rectangular hyperbola, the origin of which is at once the point at which there is no pressure of oxygen and no oxyhæmoglobin, and the curve approximates to a line representing complete saturation. If now we turn back to Fig. 22 we shall see that the curve which we have shown as representing the relation of the pressure of oxygen to the percentage of oxyhæmoglobin is identical with the curve we have just given, and therefore the law of mass action is to this extent satisfied.

Yet this satisfactory result was not reached without a struggle. The ease with which it can be demonstrated at the present time offers a very pleasant contrast to the tiresomeness of the path trod before the point of vantage now attained, had been reached.

The history of the subject forms an interesting commentary upon the psychology of research. The law of mass action was first quantitatively applied to the reaction

$$\text{Hb} + \text{O}_2 \rightleftarrows \text{HbO}_2$$

by Hüfner[1], who quite unjustifiably assumed the applicability of the law to the reaction in the form in which we have given it above and obtained a curve very similar to the one which is represented from entirely theoretical considerations.

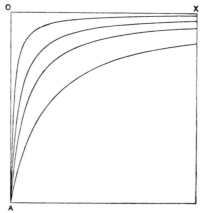

FIG. 25. Shows a series of rectangular hyperbolæ, each with A as its origin, and approximating to OX.

You can have any number of rectangular hyperbolæ all of which pass through the point A and approximate to OX, such as are shown in Fig. 25: these all satisfy the condition stated above,

$$\left(p + \frac{1}{K}\right) C_R = \frac{100}{K}.$$

The difference between them lies in the value of K. Now Hüfner assumed the correctness of the equation and set out to find the value of K. This can be done from one point. He used a number of samples of hæmoglobin prepared in different ways, determined a point for each, found the value of K, averaged these values and produced a curve. But a Nemesis awaited Hüfner. His speculations fell in the hands of a physiologist of a diametrically opposite school. Bohr(2) had inherited a tradition from the great laboratory of Ludwig which, though it may carry its holders to excessive lengths, at least forms a useful corrective to unjustifiable generalisations. Bohr's motto was that every experiment had a value, nothing which was obtained as the result of a test in the laboratory was set aside on the ground of its inherent unlikelihood or of its failure to fit general principles. Bohr therefore determined to map out the curve relating the pressure of oxygen to the relative quantities of oxy- and reduced hæmoglobin point by point, irrespective of laws, and to find out experimentally what it actually was like.

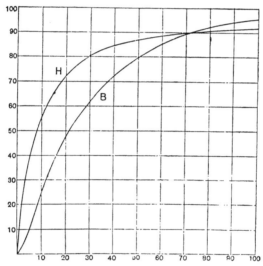

FIG. 26. Dissociation curves of hæmoglobin. *H* according to Hüfner. *B* according to Bohr.

Fig. 26 represents the curves of Bohr and Hüfner respectively; it shows that the actual curve differs fundamentally from Hüfner's, not only in the fact that it crosses it and therefore cannot be a hyperbola but that it has a double contour and consequently is not a curve of the same order at all.

At the present time it is scarcely necessary to dwell on the theory which Bohr propounded to explain his curve, quite briefly it was that when oxygen broke from hæmoglobin, the hæmoglobin itself split into globin and something rather like hæmatin which he called hæmochrome. Another explanation of this curve will be alluded to in another place. The whole question took on a new aspect when it became clear, as will appear hereafter, that the affinity of hæmoglobin for oxygen is profoundly influenced by the nature of electrolytes[3] in the solution.

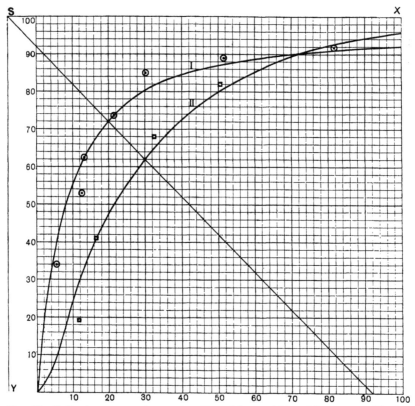

FIG. 27. Ordinates = percentage saturation of hæmoglobin with oxygen. Abscissæ = tension of oxygen in mm. of mercury. Curve I = rectangular hyperbola. $XY = 800$. Curve II = Bohr's dissociation curve of hæmoglobin.

⊙ Points determined from dialysed solution.
□ Points determined from undialysed solution.

The bearing of this discovery was at once grasped by Ff. Roberts[4], who suggested making a solution after the method of Bohr[1] and then dialysing a portion of the solution to get rid of such residual salts and traces of ether as might be in it; finally comparing the dissociation curves obtained from the dialysed and undialysed portions.

[1] I.e. precipitating the crystals with ether from centrifugalised corpuscles, washing them, redissolving them and shaking out the ether.

The experiment was performed on a solution obtained after three days' dialysis in an aseptic dialyser; this was free from the characteristic smell which always clung to our preparation of dog's hæmoglobin made by Bohr's method, it was quite neutral in reaction and its freedom from salts was kindly determined for us by Hardy, who showed that in saline concentration it was equivalent to a ·004 N solution of sodium chloride. The points on the dissociation curves of the two solutions were then determined, and are shown in Fig. 27. The round points are those of the dialysed solution, the square ones those of the undialysed solution. It was at once apparent that the latter were in very close agreement with the curve published by Bohr (denoted by II in the diagram), whilst the former fell so nearly on the rectangular hyperbola (I) as to make it in the highest degree probable that had the salts been entirely eliminated the coincidence would have been complete.

The position in 1914 was then that a dialysed solution of hæmoglobin of not very great concentration *approximated to* the hyperbolic form, but did not actually reach it. That seemed a great advance, but it was not really satisfactory to be so near finality without actually getting there. From that point the trend of events seemed rather to go in the direction of showing that the mother curve from which all those of the hæmoglobin family were derived was not a rectangular hyperbola. In collaboration with Miss Nora Tweedy (now Mrs Edkins) some hæmoglobin was investigated, of much greater purity than that used by Roberts and myself and also of much greater concentration. The dissociation curve was definitely further from the hyperbolic form than the earlier one. Adolf and Ferry[5] had the same experience, as also had Adair and I[6] later. All this time the "urge" had been to obtain solutions of maximum concentration. Adair[7] it was who first cut away from the tradition of strong hæmoglobin solutions, affirming that hæmoglobin, in its most primitive condition, would be found in dilute solutions. For such, however, the ordinary methods of gas analysis are useless. It was therefore a happy coincidence that Hartridge and Roughton[8] had adapted the reversion spectroscope—which had been invented to investigate the equilibrium between the four substances oxyhæmoglobin, carboxyhæmoglobin, oxygen and carbon monoxide—to the study of the equilibria between reduced hæmoglobin, oxyhæmoglobin and oxygen and also to that between reduced hæmoglobin, carboxyhæmoglobin and carbon monoxide. By the use of

this new technique it is possible to determine the equilibrium curve
of the system, O_2-hæmoglobin, reduced hæmoglobin and oxygen, on
solutions of a quite dilute order—such for instance as might contain
hæmoglobin in the concentration of one in one thousand.

Roughton (see Fig. 28) determined some points on this curve.
The method is not very reliable except at such points on the curve
as involve a considerable quantity both of oxy- and of reduced
hæmoglobin in the mixture—say between the limits of 30 per cent.
O_2Hb with 70 per cent. Hb and 70 per cent. O_2Hb with 30 per cent.

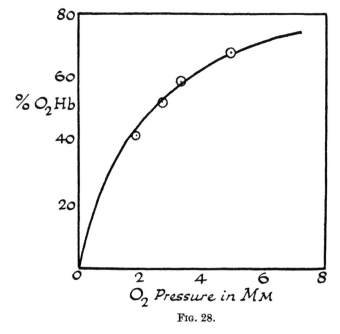

FIG. 28.

Hb. Over this region of the curve it is clear that Hartridge and
Roughton's[9] points are as nearly as may be on a rectangular hyperbola. But also it is clear that a curve which was far removed from
being hyperbolic could be drawn through the points without greater
error than the hyperbola. Moreover, the really crucial points are not
those in the middle of the curve.

It was of course impossible to leave a matter so important as the
fundamental character of the oxygen dissociation curve in so un-
satisfactory a state. Dr Selig Hecht and I[10] therefore evolved a
very simple technique for the purpose of studying the dissociation

curve. In this case it was not the curve of the reaction

$$O_2 + Hb \rightleftharpoons HbO_2,$$

but the analogous curve of the reaction

$$CO + Hb \rightleftharpoons HbCO.$$

We had a series of saturators of very different size, the smallest having a capacity of about 25 c.c., the largest of about 5 litres. Each was filled with hydrogen rigorously freed from oxygen and contained no carbon monoxide. Into each saturator was placed 5 c.c. of a solution

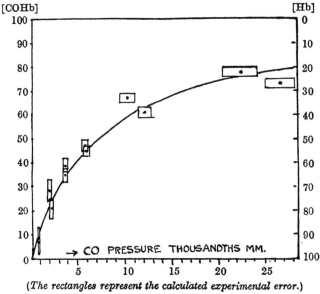

(*The rectangles represent the calculated experimental error.*)

FIG. 29.

of carboxyhæmoglobin of known CO capacity. The whole quantity of CO introduced into the saturator was therefore known with accuracy. The saturator was then shaken violently. Carbon monoxide escaped from the solution of carboxyhæmoglobin and accumulated in the atmosphere until the point was reached at which the solution and the atmosphere in contact with it were in equilibrium. After this point had been reached, a portion of the resultant mixture of carboxy-hæmoglobin and reduced hæmoglobin was withdrawn into a small vessel: here the reduced hæmoglobin became oxygenated without appreciable loss of CO by the carboxyhæmoglobin. It only remained to estimate the percentage of CO-hæmoglobin in the mixture to give all the information required. Of the total hæmoglobin present the ratio of $\dfrac{\text{COHb}}{\text{O}_2\text{Hb}}$ was the same as that of $\dfrac{\text{COHb}}{\text{Hb}}$ in the fluid contained in the tonometer, and hence we obtain the position of the point on the curve relative to the ordinate, whilst the CO pressure is easily calculated from a knowledge of (1) the volume of the saturator, (2) the amount of COHb broken down.

In the preliminary experiments of the series the estimation of the $\dfrac{\text{COHb}}{\text{O}_2\text{Hb}}$ was made with the Hartridge reversion spectroscope, with the result shown in Fig. 29 for sheep's blood.

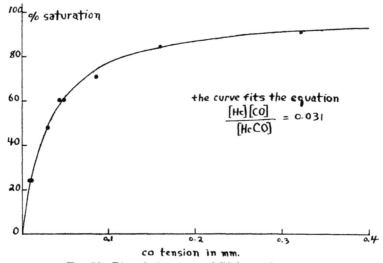

FIG. 30. Dissociation curve of CO-hæmochromogen.

Since that time more accurate methods for the estimation of the CO-hæmoglobin have been introduced, replacing the reversion spectroscope by a photographic method. This method has been found by Hecht and Morgan [11], and later by Forbes, to give a hyperbola on occasions, but not always. Therefore as things stand the hyperbola has certainly been obtained and a curve of so definite a shape cannot be obtained repeatedly, by chance, using accurate methods. It must be assumed therefore that on certain occasions the curve really did assume the hyperbolic form, though on other occasions it as certainly did not. The cause of the difference is unknown, but experience showed that the longer the solution was kept, even though it was kept under quite rigid conditions at $-1°$ C., the more closely would the curve derived from it be to the hyperbola—and that is a curious thing!

That seems to be the position as regards dilute hæmoglobin solutions; really concentrated ones never seem to give the hyperbola.

Carbon monoxide forms a reversible compound with hæmochromogen, the dissociation curve of which has been studied by Anson and Mirsky [12]. They found it to be definitely a rectangular hyperbola, the hæmochromogen being 50 per cent. saturated at $37°$ C. when exposed to a pressure of carbon monoxide of $\frac{31}{1000}$ mm. (see Fig. 30).

If then we may regard the fundamental difference between hæmochromogen and hæmoglobin as being the different condition in which the globin is found in the two substances, we should be directed towards the conclusion that where the protein is in the denatured state the curve is a hyperbola, and in so far as the curve differs from the hyperbola in the case of hæmoglobin the difference is imposed by the protein.

We have yet to learn the molecular weight of hæmochromogen and it may be much less than that of hæmoglobin, a difference which also might influence the shape of the curve.

The important point is that the most primitive dissociation curve of which we know, that from which the other curves appear to be derived, is indeed a hyperbola.

REFERENCES

(1) Hüfner. *Arch. f. Anat. u. Physiol.* v. 187. 1901.

(2) Bohr. *Zentralb. f. Physiol.* xvii. 682. 1879.

(3) Barcroft and Camis. *Journ. Physiol.* xxxix. 118. 1909.

(4) Barcroft and Roberts. *Journ. Physiol.* xxxix. 143. 1909.

(5) Adolf and Ferry. *Journ. Biol. Chem.* xlvii. 547. 1921.

(6) Adair, Barcroft and Bock. *Journ. Physiol.* lv. 332. 1921.

(7) Adair. Fellowship Dissertation presented to King's College, Cambridge, 1921.

(8) Hartridge and Roughton. *Proc. Roy. Soc.* A. civ. 398. 1923.

(9) Hartridge and Roughton. *Proc. Roy. Soc.* A. cvii. 673. 1925.

(10) Barcroft. *Journ. Chem. Soc.* cxxix. 1146. May, 1926.

(11) Hecht and Morgan. In press.

(12) Anson and Mirsky. *Journ. Physiol.* lx. 63. 1925.

CHAPTER XI

THE DISSOCIATION CURVE OF HÆMOGLOBIN
(continued)

THE further consideration of the graphic representations defining the equilibrium which exists between oxygen, reduced hæmoglobin and oxyhæmoglobin must start, in the present state of knowledge, from two assumptions: (1) that the molecular weight of hæmoglobin is of the order of 70,000, each molecule uniting reversibly with four oxygen or CO molecules, and (2) that the basal curve from which others are derived is the hyperbola; even though we are driven back to CO-hæmochromogen in order to be certain of finding it.

What then is the shape of the curve which represents a reversible reaction between one molecule of hæmoglobin and four of oxygen? The answer is not quite simple, because the form of the curve cannot be stated until another matter is settled. Do the molecules of oxygen unite with the hæmoglobin molecule one by one, or do they join in the "all-or-none" principle? In the first case the reaction would be

$$Hb_4{}^1 \; + O_2 \rightleftharpoons Hb_4O_2,$$
$$Hb_4O_2 + O_2 \rightleftharpoons Hb_4O_4,$$
$$Hb_4O_4 + O_2 \rightleftharpoons Hb_4O_6,$$
$$Hb_4O_6 + O_2 \rightleftharpoons Hb_4O_8.$$

In the second case the reaction would simply be

$$Hb_4 + 4O_2 \rightleftharpoons Hb_4O_8.$$

In the last case any molecule which is stable must be either Hb_4 or Hb_4O_8; the intermediate molecules may be formed, but if so they are less stable than those in reduced and fully oxidised molecules and therefore cannot remain in their presence.

On general grounds it is much more likely that the oxygen molecules join seriatim. On the other hand no one has ever isolated, or even discovered cogent evidence of the existence of, the bodies Hb_4O_2, Hb_4O_4 and Hb_4O_6.

But to return to the curves, what sort of curves depict the mathematical representation of these two alternative forms of reaction?

---

[1] By Hb_4 is meant four hæmatins attached probably to one globin.

Taking first that in which the oxygen molecules join one by one, if each oxygen molecule is entirely uninfluenced by its fellows and so far away from them as to be quite independent, the curve which represents each of the four constituent reactions will be a rectangular hyperbola and the curve which represents the whole four will be a hyperbola also. Written after the notation introduced by A. V. Hill[1], if x be the oxygen pressure, y the percentage of the whole hæmoglobin which is oxyhæmoglobin and K the equilibrium constant,

$$\frac{y}{100} = \frac{Kx}{1 + Kx}.$$

If on the other hand the intermediate oxides are so unstable as to be incapable of persisting, the reaction would be represented by the equation

$$\frac{y}{100} = \frac{Kx^4}{1 + Kx^4}.$$

The curve which represents the last equation is not a hyperbola, but one with a large inflection. (See fig. 31.)

As Adair has pointed out, if we are not prepared to make either the assumption that the oxygen molecules are quite independent on the one hand, or, on the other, that their union is absolutely dependent upon one another, but that each oxygen atom, as it joins, reduces the affinity of the whole molecule for the next, we could assume a curve with some degree of inflection but intermediate between those given in Fig. 31. As a matter of experience, curves of this kind have usually been obtained when dilute hæmoglobin has been equilibrated long enough with carbon monoxide for the purpose. But although much pains have been spent on this reaction it may be doubted whether any finality has been reached as yet. As so often occurs when hæmoglobin is the object of investigation we seem to be "between the devil and the deep sea." Clearly a dilute solution of hæmoglobin is in theory the proper one to study; on the other hand all experience shows that such a solution is extremely labile. Douglas, Haldane and Haldane[2] emphasised the ease with which hæmoglobin is destroyed when shaken in dilute solution, and recommended the addition of ammonia in small quantities. Undoubtedly in slightly alkaline solution the globin shows much less tendency to coagulate than in neutral ones, nevertheless at best the hæmoglobin is not very stable. It is the opinion of Roughton, who has great experience on this particular point, that hæmoglobin in dilute solution cannot be trusted to stand the amount of shaking and general maltreatment which is required for the establishment of an equilibrium between it and the very low concentrations of carbon monoxide used on such occasions. Evidence can be obtained as to the general nature of the reaction with the establishment of an equilibrium by the study of the velocity of the reactions between

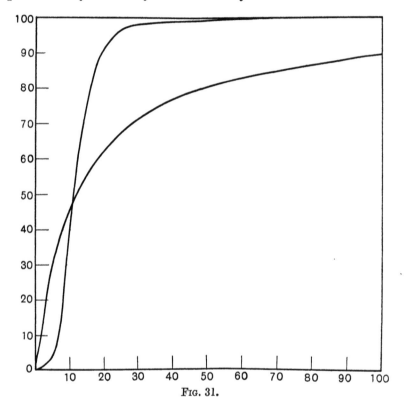

FIG. 31.

hæmoglobin and carbon monoxide or oxygen. Such evidence will be discussed in Chapters XIV and XV. Meanwhile we can do little more than make a list of the conditions which influence the equilibrium.

The dissociation curve of oxyhæmoglobin may be influenced by any of the following conditions: (1) temperature, (2) saline concentration of the solvent, (3) hydrogen-ion concentration, (4) concentration of the hæmoglobin itself.

The effect of temperature may be taken first because probably it alters the curve in a very simple way. The point is an important one, so I shall pause for a moment to consider it. Imagine the curve drawn on a sheet of india-rubber, which could be stretched horizontally without alteration in its vertical dimensions; then the alteration in the curve which would be caused by rise of temperature could be simulated by mere stretching of the sheet. This relationship is excellently shown in the series of curves given by A. V. Hill and Brown(3) for blood at different temperatures. They are as it were all the same curve but drawn on different horizontal scales. The property is such as would be caused by a simple alteration in the equilibrium constant of the reaction, without any alteration in such factors as are responsible for the degree of inflection of the curves. Therefore we at once get at a conception which separates causes which define the curve into two categories, those which are responsible for the equilibrium constant and for the degree of inflection respectively. A particular factor may affect both the constant and the inflection but it need not necessarily do so and temperature appears to affect the former without altering the latter. The effect of temperature will, however, be treated in greater detail in a future chapter.

The effect of salts. Concerning the effect of salts on the oxygen dissociation curve we know very little. Among the earliest observations made by Camis and myself(4) was the one that certain salts added to a solution of hæmoglobin in distilled water altered the curve, making it more inflected. I never know whether it was more fortunate or unfortunate that the observation was made at so early a stage; it was unfortunate because at that time the effect of hydrogen-ion concentration was not appreciated and therefore not controlled and it is certain that many of the salts used, e.g. sodium phosphate, altered the hydrogen-ion concentration of the fluid. Moreover, the distilled-water solution was not itself so free from salts as it would have been, had the investigation been made a year later. The fortunate circumstance, however, was that had the discovery not been made at the time it was, it might have been long postponed; for the whole effect of salts on the dissociation curve might have been attributed to changes in hydrogen-ion concentration. In any case the thing must be done again and it wants doing both in relation to the hydrogen-ion concentration and the hæmoglobin concentration. We are only waiting for a certain base line from which to start, in order to test the effect of salts on dilute solutions of hæmoglobin. So far as may be gathered from the work on the velocity constants carried out by Hartridge and Roughton(5) salts have no effect on the rate at which really dilute solutions (say of the order of one part of hæmoglobin to 1000 of water) take up or give out oxygen. The work of Adair (6), however, shows that the osmotic pressure of the hæmoglobin does depend upon the saline content of the solution in which it is dissolved; above a certain saline

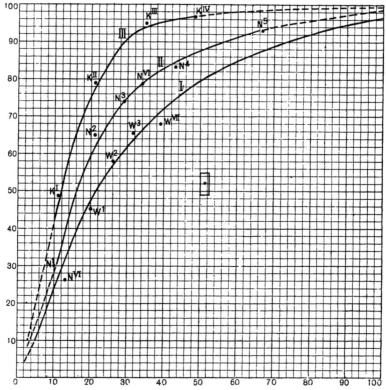

FIG. 32. Ordinate = percentage saturation of hæmoglobin. Abscissa = tension of oxygen in mm. of mercury.

  I. Dissociation curve of hæmoglobin dissolved in water.
  II. ,,   ,,   ,,   ·7 per cent. NaCl.
  III. ,,   ,,   ,,   ·9 per cent. KCl.
  Rectangle surrounding point = magnitude of experimental error. Temperature 37–38° C.

content the osmotic pressure is stable over a large range. Stabilisation of the osmotic pressure likely enough means stabilisation of the degree of inflection of the oxygen dissociation curve.

The effect of hydrogen-ion concentration. It will clear the ground to commence by saying that, so far as is known, the effect of carbonic acid on hæmoglobin is not specific but is due to alteration of the hydrogen-ion concentration of the solution. The proof as obtained by Cecil Murray and myself of this is as follows:

Starting from the known facts that the effect of carbonic acid is to reduce the affinity of hæmoglobin for oxygen, and that the effect of increased hydrogen-ion concentration is qualitatively the same, if CO_2 owes its effect simply to the incidental accumulation of hydrogen ions a given hæmoglobin solution of a given cH should have the same affinity for oxygen, whether that concentration of hydrogen ions be established by the addition of CO_2 or of any other acid. This of course assumes that the solutions are similar in all other

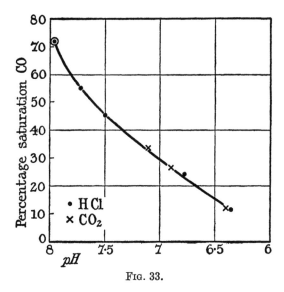

FIG. 33.

respects. To put the matter in another way, if a solution of hæmoglobin be taken and divided into two portions, and if in the case of one portion a number of points be determined in which (a) the percentage saturation of oxygen at a known oxygen pressure is plotted against (b) the cH (or pH)—the cH being altered by the addition of HCl—and if in the case of the other portion a similar curve be drawn, but with the cH regulated by exposure to CO_2, then if CO_2 affects the affinity for oxygen merely by establishing a certain hydrogen-ion concentration, and if HCl does the same, the two curves should be superposable.

Fig. 33 illustrates the results of such an experiment (7). The gas to which the hæmoglobin was exposed was not oxygen but carbon monoxide; so that the equilibrium under consideration was not

$$Hb + O_2 = HbO_2,$$

but $$Hb + CO = HbCO.$$

The latter, however, is supposed to observe the same general laws as the former, though the concentration of carbon monoxide necessary to produce a given percentage saturation of HbCO is of course much lower than that of oxygen necessary to produce the same percentage of oxyhæmoglobin.

The reason for not using oxyhæmoglobin was that the hydrogen-ion concentration of mixtures of oxy- and reduced hæmoglobins is, or was at the time when these observations were carried out, beyond the known powers of the platinum electrode.

In each case the concentration of CO to which hæmoglobin was exposed was the same, but the more acid the solution, the lower the percentage saturation with CO. The following table gives (1) the percentage saturation, (2) the acid by addition of which the reaction was adjusted, and (3) the hydrogen-ion concentration resulting.

Observation	1	2	3	4	5	6	7	8
Percentage saturation when exposed to 0·01 % CO in H_2	72	55	45	33	26	24	12	12
Acid used for regulating pH	None	?	HCl	CO_2	CO_2	HCl	CO_2	HCl
pH of solution	7·96	7·73	7·50	7·10	6·90	6·82	6·39	6·36

Adair[8] has published a set of curves, each of which represents the equilibrium between oxygen and human hæmoglobin at a given hydrogen-ion concentration. The hydrogen-ion concentrations vary from $10^{-8} \times \cdot 8$ (pH 8·3) to $10^{-8} \times 100$ (pH 6·0).

The hæmoglobin was dialysed first against water which contained CO_2, so as to detach the sodium from the hæmoglobin (this was done with different degrees of thoroughness, accounting for the differing hydrogen-ion concentrations), and the hæmoglobin was subsequently dialysed against distilled water to eliminate the carbonic acid. The curves are given in Fig. 34. A similar series of curves was published by Means and myself[9] in 1913, representing the effect of carbonic acid on the dissociation curve of hæmoglobin.

At first sight these curves look rather confused, the fact being that the first few millimetres of CO_2 seemed to alter the degree of inflection very much; as the hydrogen-ion concentration increased the inflection became relatively constant, the CO_2 affecting the curves much in the way that temperature might do.

Thus the first effect, when CO_2 is added to a salt-free or nearly salt-free solution of hæmoglobin, includes a salt effect. Herein hæmoglobin differs from blood. CO_2 has no effect or almost no effect on the degree of inflection of the oxygen dissociation curve of blood, the inflection is already present even in the CO_2-free blood, being apparently produced and stabilised by the salts; the effect of concentration we do not yet know. The curves published by Bohr, Hasselbalch

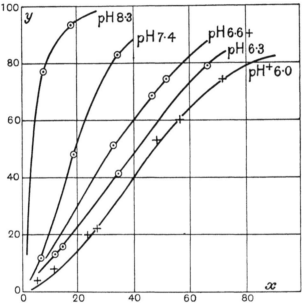

FIG. 34. Oxygen dissociation curves at different H-ion concentrations.
y = percentage of oxygenation.
x = oxygen pressure in mm.

and Krogh [10] and Barcroft and Poulton [11], as well as by Douglas, Haldane and Haldane [12], illustrating the effect of CO_2 on blood exposed to CO in the absence of oxygen, all agree in showing that there is very little difference in the degree of inflection of the curves at various CO_2 pressures. The curve for any one CO_2 pressure, for blood, could be almost superposed on that for any other pressure by merely altering the horizontal scale on which it is drawn.

The degree to which the curves (at varying CO_2 pressures) are unaltered in inflection may be shown by a comparison of Figs. 35

and 36. Fig. 35 is a reproduction of Douglas, Haldane and Haldane's
original graph representing the equilibrium between CO and blood
at varying CO_2 pressures. The curves are drawn freehand without
reference to any theory. Fig. 36 shows the same experimental points
referred to a series of lines of equal inflection. [Note that at 30 per cent.

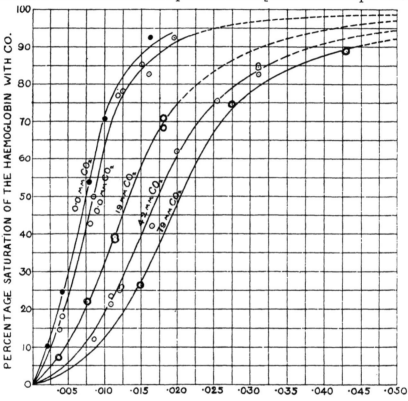

PRESSURE OF CO IN PERCENTAGE OF ONE ATMOSPHERE.

FIG. 35. Dissociation curves of CO-hæmoglobin in absence of oxygen, at 38° C., and
with various pressures of CO_2. ○ blood of Douglas. ⊙ blood of Haldane.

saturation on the 0 mm. CO_2 line the pressure of CO is ·042 mm. and
on the 79 mm. line at the same saturation the pressure is ·105, and the

ratio of $\dfrac{·042}{·105} = ·4$; the corresponding pressures at 70 per cent.

saturation ·086 and ·21, ratio $\dfrac{·086}{·21} = ·4$, and so on.]

Accepting the view that carbonic acid has no specific action
on hæmoglobin, i.e. that it does not replace oxygen directly after

the manner of CO, but that its action is indirect by producing a change in the hydrogen-ion concentration of the fluid, the further question must be asked: In virtue of what mechanism does an increase of the hydrogen-ion concentration of the hæmoglobin solution weaken the bond between hæmoglobin and oxygen, and alternatively,

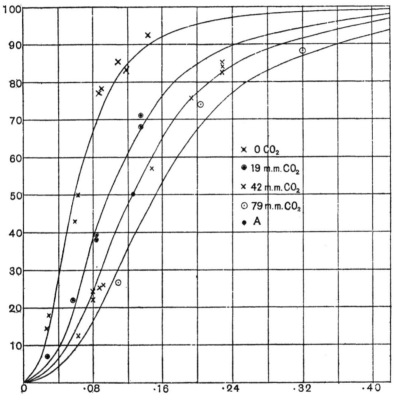

FIG. 36. Dissociation curves of CO-hæmoglobin. Curves drawn from formula

$$y/100 = \frac{Kx^n}{1 + Kx^n}.$$

The curve is based on the coincidence of point A with the corresponding point on Fig. 35.

Ordinate = percentage saturation with CO.
Abscissa = CO pressure in mm. Points indicated are the determinations of Haldane and Douglas.

by what process does a reduction in hydrogen-ion concentration strengthen the bond between oxygen and hæmoglobin?

This enquiry has been pursued by A. V. Hill[13], [14], [15] and his colleagues, and also by L. J. Henderson[16], [17] on the theoretical side, and against it has been directed the whole artillery of the Rockefeller Institute by Dr Van Slyke[18], [19], [20].

There seems to be general agreement on one point, namely, that the key of the situation lies in the fact of oxyhæmoglobin being a stronger acid than reduced hæmoglobin. This has been shown to be the case by Parsons[21], who made actual hydrogen-ion measurements of oxygenated and reduced blood under similar conditions and found that the fact of oxygenating the blood (or alternatively treating it with carbon monoxide) increased the hydrogen-ion concentration by about 8 per cent. Imagine then a solution containing reduced hæmoglobin, CO_2 and Na; some of the Na will be united with the CO_2 and some with the hæmoglobin. Some such crude scheme as the following may be pictured:

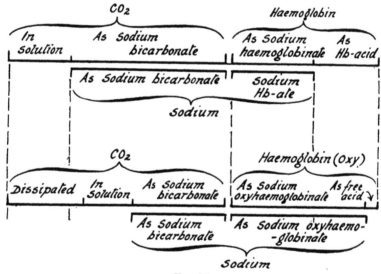

FIG. 37.

The CO_2 is present in two forms, partly in solution and partly united with the sodium. The reduced hæmoglobin similarly is present partly as the free acid and partly as the sodium salt; thus a certain quantity of sodium is united with the CO_2 and a certain quantity with the reduced hæmoglobin. These facts are indicated in the upper scheme. Suppose now that the reduced hæmoglobin becomes oxidised, the sodium will, so to speak, be pulled in the direction of the hæmoglobin, and therefore less sodium will unite with the CO_2, a greater quantity of CO_2 will go into solution and, if the solution had previously been in equilibrium with the atmosphere, CO_2 will be driven off. If CO_2 be put into the solution the whole chain of events will shift in the opposite direction.

It now remains to discuss more completely the possible mechanism by which increased hydrogen-ion concentration affects the oxygen-binding power of the hæmoglobin. No doubt in a complex agglomeration of amino-acids such as make up the protein molecule, there are many hydrogen ions which can be replaced by sodium—just how many, has been a matter of some dispute: but Henderson and Hill are in agreement in supposing that not all these are of equal value in affecting the affinity of hæmoglobin for oxygen. Henderson[16] supposes that for each molecule of oxygen there is one particular hydrogen ion, situated in a special position in the protein molecule, near to where the hæmatin and the protein join; which ion is the only one affecting the oxygen-binding power. Hill[14], [15] has suggested as an expansion of his theory that in the molecule of hæmoglobin, $(Hb)_n$, there is only one relevant hydrogen ion for n molecules of dissociable oxygen. If that atom be replaced by base, the hæmoglobin unites with oxygen much more readily than if the critical hydrogen ion is itself present.

The theories of Hill and Henderson may account for the fact that the curves for hæmoglobin which Means and I obtained are much less spread out than those for blood; it seems doubtful whether in the absence of base, hydrogen-ion concentration would have any effect at all on the affinity of hæmoglobin for oxygen. The solution used by Means and myself[9] certainly contained very little base as compared with blood.

It is doubtful whether we can speculate further on this subject with profit. It will be shown later that in any case it is only in a certain range of hydrogen-ion concentration that the characteristic effect is found. In solutions more acid than $pH = 5\cdot5$ and more alkaline than $pH = 7\cdot6$ it does not exist.

The mention of one particular hydrogen ion being on a different level of importance from the rest raises the question of counting the number of free hydrogen ions which exist in the hæmoglobin molecule. This estimation has been carried out by various observers, Straub[22], Parsons[23], A. V. Hill[14], Adair[24] and others, but most recently the matter has been gone into with great detail and thoroughness at the Rockefeller Institute in New York. The following calculations, which are based by Adair on the data of Hastings, Sendroy, Murray and Heidelberger[20], assume that the isoelectric point of horse hæmoglobin is pH 6·78, at lower pH the hæmoglobin acts as a base and at higher pH it acts as an acid. Further, it is assumed that the molecule of hæmoglobin contains four equivalents of iron.

The table gives the number of equivalents of acid (italics) or alkali (block type) which one molecule (mol. wt. about 70,000) unites with at the pH stated.

pH	6·0	6·6	6·78	7·0	7·4	7·8	8·0	8·3	9·0	9·5
Combined acid or base	*5·56*	*1·32*	0·00	1·9	5·9	10·1	11·8	14·2	18·2	20·4

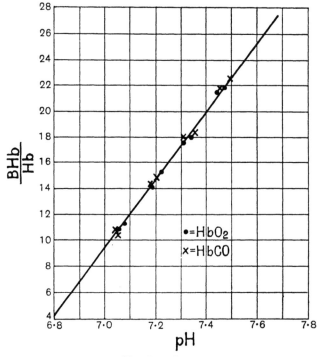

FIG. 38. (See text.)

It may here be specially noted that the figures given are for horse hæmoglobin only, and would be somewhat different for the hæmoglobins of other animals—another instance of the specificity of hæmoglobin.

I spoke of Fig. 37 as a crude presentation of the facts. Its crudity may suitably be compared with the very beautiful quantitative statement from the Rockefeller Institute of the relative quantities of

Hb-acid and sodium hæmoglobinate which exist at any particular degree of acidity of the fluid. Fig. 38 shows as the ordinate the quantity of hæmoglobin united to base (BHb) in proportion to that not so united (Hb) and as the abscissa the *p*H. It will be seen moreover that the graph is equally true whether the hæmoglobin is in the form of oxy- or CO-Hb—a point which will be considered in Chapter XIV.

REFERENCES

(1) HILL, A. V. *Journ. Physiol.* XL. iv. 1910.

(2) DOUGLAS, HALDANE AND HALDANE. *Journ. Physiol.* XLIV. 281. 1912.

(3) BROWN, W. E. L. AND HILL, A. V. *Proc. Roy. Soc.* B. XCIV. 307. 1923.

(4) BARCROFT AND CAMIS. *Journ. Physiol.* XXXIX. 118. 1909.

(5) HARTRIDGE AND ROUGHTON. *Proc. Roy. Soc.* A. CVII. 677. 1925.

(6) ADAIR quoted by BARCROFT. *Journ. Chem. Soc.* CXXIX. 1169. May, 1926.

(7) BARCROFT AND MURRAY. *Phil. Trans. Roy. Soc.* B. CCXI. 465. 1922.

(8) ADAIR, BOCK AND FIELD. *Journ. Biol. Chem.* LXIII. 505 and 537. 1925.

(9) BARCROFT AND MEANS. *Journ. Physiol.* XLVII. xxvii. 1913.

(10) BOHR, HASSELBALCH AND KROGH. *Skand. Archiv f. Physiol.* XVI. 409. 1904.

(11) BARCROFT AND POULTON. *Journ. Physiol.* XLVI. iv. 1913.

(12) DOUGLAS, HALDANE AND HALDANE. *Journ. Physiol.* XLIV. 287. 1912.

(13) HILL, A. V. *Biochem. Journ.* XV. 583. 1921.

(14) HILL, A. V. *Journ. Biol. Chem.* LI. 359. 1922.

(15) BROWN, W. E. L. AND HILL, A. V. *Proc. Roy. Soc.* B. XCIV. 326. 1923.

(16) HENDERSON, L. J. *Journ. Biol. Chem.* XLI. 401. 1920.

(17) HENDERSON, L. J. *Certain Aspects of Biochemistry*, p. 175. 1926.

(18) VAN SLYKE, HASTINGS, HEIDELBERGER AND NEILL. *Journ. Biol. Chem.* LIV. 447. 1922.

(19) HASTINGS, VAN SLYKE, NEILL, HEIDELBERGER AND HARINGTON. *Journ. Biol. Chem.* LX. 89. 1924.

(20) HASTINGS, SENDROY, MURRAY AND HEIDELBERGER. *Journ. Biol. Chem.* LXI. 317. 1924.

(21) PARSONS. *Journ. Physiol.* LI. 440. 1917.

(22) STRAUB AND MEIER. *Biochem. Zeitsch.* XC. 305. 1918.

(23) PARSONS. *Journ. Physiol.* LVI. 1. 1922.

(24) ADAIR, BOCK AND FIELD. *Journ. Biol. Chem.* LXIII. 517. 1925.

CHAPTER XII

THEORIES OF THE UNION OF OXYGEN WITH HÆMOGLOBIN

To say that every worker on hæmoglobin has had a pet theory of the way in which that substance unites with oxygen would of course be a gross exaggeration, nevertheless the lure of this subject has been remarkable—perhaps "remarkable" is the wrong word because the importance of the subject is so great. After all, biologically, the re-action is one upon which much of life depends and, biochemically, there is much to be learned about proteins in general from a complete understanding of hæmoglobin. Let us say that the lure of the subject has been "more than considerable."

When *The Respiratory Function of the Blood* was first written, interest centred largely about the question of whether the union of oxygen with hæmoglobin was a chemical or a physical one. Of the seven theories that come to the mind six are chemical and one is physical. In so far as there is any real difference between a chemical and physical conception, there seems to be no doubt that oxyhæmoglobin is a true chemical compound.

At the risk perhaps of some repetition let us state the case for and against the adsorption hypothesis. This theory was put forward by Wolfgang Ostwald (1) at a time when the idea of adsorption was very much in the air. The underlying conception was that the large hæmo-globin molecule attracted oxygen molecules to it which remained adherent to the surface in view of their electrical charges. It assumed that the hæmoglobin molecule was something large enough to have a surface with definite properties as opposed to those of the rest of the molecule, and that the quantity of oxygen which adhered to the surface at any given time depended upon the pressure of oxygen present and could be increased indefinitely by increasing the oxygen pressure. Of course it is not suggested that equal increments of pressure produce equal increments in the quantity of adsorbed oxygen. The relation is a parabolic one.

The actual facts are in conflict with the above statement of theory at several points, brief and crude as that statement may be.

In the first place the relation between hæmoglobin and oxygen is definitely not a parabolic one as is attested by the multitude of dissociation curves which have been determined. Of these, most present definitely a double inflection, some appear not to do so, but none is of the shape depicted by Ostwald. One is tempted to ask why he should ever have published curves which appear to be so widely divorced from experimental truth. The reason is simple enough: at the time when Ostwald's paper was written there was very little exact knowledge as to the shape of the oxygen dissociation curve.

The contention that hæmoglobin can unite with an indefinitely large quantity of oxygen appears also to be contrary to the facts as determined experimentally. The same is true of carbon monoxide. If blood is brought into equilibrium with oxygen in the cold at atmospheric pressure, the hæmoglobin will not absorb an appreciably greater quantity of oxygen even if exposed to an atmosphere of pure oxygen gas. The dissociation curve has become asymptotic.

The same thing has been shown with regard to the affinity of carbon monoxide for hæmoglobin, and in this case the demonstration is much more striking than in the case of oxygen because, owing to the fact that hæmoglobin has some 250[1] times as great an affinity for carbon monoxide as for oxygen, the curve becomes asymptotic at a very much lower pressure. The proof that there is a definite limit for the amount of carbon monoxide with which a given quantity of hæmoglobin will unite was shown in a very elegant way by W. E. L. Brown[2].

It is not merely that the union of oxygen and hæmoglobin obeys the law of definite proportions, but also that it obeys the law of simple proportions, as has been shown in the chapter on its specific oxygen capacity. It may be pointed out further that the quantity of oxygen with which hæmoglobin unites, namely, one gram molecular weight of oxygen to 17,000 grams of hæmoglobin, offers a conception very different from that which one ordinarily has with regard to adsorption, the latter conception being that of a large molecule with numerous small molecules adhering to its surface and having no particular preference for any one portion of the surface rather than another. In the case of hæmoglobin the 17,000-gram molecular unit unites with but one gram molecular weight of oxygen, and further this molecule attaches itself to a perfectly definite portion of the hæmoglobin molecule, namely, the hæmatin, and

[1] Sheep's blood at room temperature.

even in it the oxygen would appear to have a definite relation to the iron atom.

The whole subject has been put very well in a letter written by Neil Adam(3) to *Nature* which, with the author's permission and that of the editor of the magazine, I quote. This letter has the advantage of defining adsorption in such a way as to make it something more definite than is vaguely conceived in most people's minds.

THE COMBINATION BETWEEN OXYGEN AND HÆMOGLOBIN AND THE CRITERIA OF ADSORPTION

Hæmoglobin combines with oxygen approximately in the ratio of 16,670 to 32, by weight, as was shown by Peters (*Journal of Physiology*, vol. XLIV. p. 131). It is clear, then, that in solution the particle of hæmoglobin is very much larger than the particle of oxygen which combines with it. If one might assume that the densities and shapes of the particles were similar, then their surfaces would be in the ratio 64 to 1; in any case, and whatever the degree of aggregation of the particles, probably only a very small part of the surface of the hæmoglobin particles can be actually covered by oxygen when combination ceases at the stage of oxyhæmoglobin.

This shows that the attraction of hæmoglobin for oxygen is a highly localised property of the hæmoglobin particles. For if this attraction were more or less evenly distributed over the surface, it would be satisfied only to a small extent, when a small part of the surface was covered, and at higher concentrations of oxygen than those which are found experimentally to give saturation with oxygen, more oxygen would be taken up.

Taking the thermal motions of the particles into account does not affect this argument, since the movements of the particles according to the laws of the kinetic theory do not affect their surface areas.

Now, if the attraction of hæmoglobin for oxygen is of such a character that it is satisfied when only a small portion of the surface is covered, it seems impossible to regard this combination as a case of adsorption.

The criteria of adsorption are perhaps not yet so well defined as could be wished, if differences of opinion as to whether a given process should be classified as adsorption or not are to be avoided. I am inclined to think that a process is rightly classified as adsorption, *if the substance taken up by the surface continues to be taken up until the whole surface is uniformly covered*, but not otherwise. Covering the surface uniformly is of course meant in the sense in which a gas or homogeneous solid is said to fill space uniformly; that is, uniformly to a being armed with a microscope to which individual atoms are small.

This definition is both definite theoretically, and in accordance with common conceptions of adsorption. It is difficult, indeed, to see what other definition is possible in the present state of knowledge. It is perhaps, however, desirable to state the definition clearly; although, as I feel it must have been present, whether formulated or accepted as self-evident, to the minds of many workers on adsorption, no sort of novelty is claimed for it here.

A definition of adsorption based on the nature or quality of the forces attracting the adsorbed substance, is now impossible, since it appears proved by Langmuir's work that there is no difficulty in accounting both qualitatively and quantitatively for many cases of adsorption, by means of the already very familiar forces which cause combination between metals and oxygen to form oxides, or the forces which bring about solution.

Obviously adsorption cannot be defined as "that which occurs at the surface of a colloid"; since colloids themselves are not yet a well-defined class of substances, and indeed the best studied cases of adsorption are at plane interfaces, not at the surfaces of colloids.

With the definition of adsorption proposed, a process would be excluded if, as with hæmoglobin and oxygen, combination occurs only at some defined locality on the surface. Similarly, the ordinary reactions of organic chemistry will be excluded, as they should be, since the substances taken up go to definite atomic groupings in the molecule. The combination of oxygen with hæmoglobin is seen to belong to the same class as most organic reactions.

It remains to examine whether the definition is practically applicable to known cases of adsorption, as well as theoretically justified; and whether, in the case of oxygen and hæmoglobin, the arguments originally put forward in support of the adsorption process are cogent enough to override the definition.

All cases of adsorption, from a gaseous phase, or from solution, on plane, or nearly plane, interfaces, are obviously compatible with the definition, since the common method of calculating the amount of adsorption assumes uniformity of distribution on the surface, and the results are generally expressed per sq. cm. of interface.

In the cases of adsorption on colloidal surfaces, when the extent of surface is usually not known, and the adsorption is expressed per gram of adsorbent, the definition is probably also applicable. Mecklenburg (*Zeitsch. f. physikal. Chemie*, vol. LXXXIII. p. 622) described experiments showing in several cases that the adsorption on different specimens of the same adsorbent, prepared, however, under different conditions, varied in a precisely similar way with concentration for each adsorbent, but the total amount adsorbed per gram was proportional to a factor in each case, this factor being presumably proportional to the area of the adsorbent.

In proposing the theory that the oxygen in oxyhæmoglobin is held by adsorption, Wo. Ostwald (*Koll. Zeitsch.* vol. II. pp. 264, 294) based the argument on two supposed facts: first, that no definite saturation point of oxygen with hæmoglobin could be found, a fact now shown to be incorrect; and, second, that the amount of oxygen taken up at different pressures could be fairly accurately represented, under certain conditions, by the so-called "adsorption isotherm," $y = kc^n$ (y = amount taken up, c = concentration of oxygen).

The mere fact that the variation of the amount taken up fits the "adsorption isotherm" does not seem now to be a sufficient ground for classing a process as adsorption. The "isotherm" has, until quite recently, been an empirical fact without theoretical explanation; and not only does it contain two independent arbitrary constants, which makes the fitting of a set of experimental data easier than would be the case otherwise; but also it is, at the best, usually only accurate at low concentrations, divergencies being found at higher concentrations.

A more accurate equation relating amount adsorbed to concentration has been deduced recently (Henry, *Phil. Mag.* vol. XLIV. p. 689, 1922) on the assumptions of a small range of molecular attraction and a mono-molecular adsorbed layer, using well-established equations of the kinetic theory; and the author also gives a derivation of the "adsorption isotherm" on theoretical grounds. It would seem undesirable, however, to use the form of the relation between amount adsorbed and concentration as a criterion of adsorption, for this relation can never be a very simple conception, depending as it does on so many factors; but nothing could be simpler than to conceive of a surface as possessing either localised or diffuse attraction for a substance it takes up. It may be that in some instances it is not yet possible to form any estimate of the fraction of the surface covered; yet as accurate knowledge of the dimensions of molecules and of their orientation on surfaces accumulates, the applicability of the criterion here suggested will increase. I have tried to show, however, that it is already more generally applicable than any other.

N. K. ADAM.

The University, Sheffield, March 6.

Conant's theory. Though out of its chronological order, mention may be made here of a recent paper by Conant and Scott [4]. These authors, impressed with the view that nitrogen appears more soluble in blood than it is in the amount of water which blood contains, have revived the adsorption theory, or rather have combined it with the theory of chemical combination. In their view the inflection is caused by an increase in the concentration of the oxygen around the hæmoglobin molecule, so that at low pressures the actual pressure of oxygen in contact with the hæmoglobin is greater than the pressure throughout the fluid generally.

The evidence in favour of oxy- and carboxyhæmoglobin being chemical compounds, is in fact of just the same nature as that of any other substance which exists as the results of a balanced action. Granting then the chemical nature of the union let us turn to the theories which treat of it on a chemical basis.

Hüfner's theory [5] is the simplest of these and assumes the reaction to be a unimolecular one:

$$Hb + O_2 \rightleftharpoons HbO_2.$$

I say "assumes" advisedly because Hüfner never was at pains to prove his theory except in one respect. Though he published a dissociation curve, the curve was obtained from theory and not the theory from the curve. Hüfner never determined the curve from a series of points. He assumed that the equation was as stated and therefore that equilibrium would be represented by the equation

$$[Hb]\,[O_2] = K\,[HbO_2].$$

He then determined the value of K by averaging a great number of impossibly divergent determinations and calculated the curve. The one respect in which he tried to verify his theory was that of ascertaining whether the hæmoglobin was present in the form of single molecules. For this purpose he, in collaboration with Gansser, determined the osmotic pressure and found that it corresponded to a molecular weight of 16,670, and therefore involves but a single atom of iron in the molecule. The osmotic pressure of hæmoglobin is the subject of another chapter; how Hüfner and Gansser managed to obtain the figure for it, which agreed so well with their theory, must remain for ever a mystery.

Bohr's theory (6). Bohr approached the matter from a standpoint precisely opposite to that of Hüfner. He determined a dissociation curve with great accuracy, and then tried to fit an equation based upon some theoretical reasoning to the curve. The theory which yielded, to him, a satisfactory solution was as follows: hæmoglobin consists of two substances united together, the protein and the iron-containing part, which he called "hæmochrome." When oxy-hæmoglobin was formed the oxygen broke up the combination dissociating the hæmochrome from the globin. Thus a double decomposition took place.

There is no further evidence for Bohr's theory than that which he adduced, namely, that with its aid you can draw a curve which coincides very closely with the one he determined. No attempt has, as far as I know, been made to stretch the theory so as to include the great number of curves which have since been brought to light under different circumstances. Possibly such an attempt could be made with success if one assumed that the affinity of the "hæmochrome for the oxygen" varied with the conditions, being very great in circumstances under which the curve approached most nearly to a hyperbola, so that under such conditions there was little or no dissociation of the pigment from the globin.

Hill's theory (7), (8). It is natural that all theories should reflect the times in which they are deduced. Whether or not they stand the test of time depends in a measure on whether the knowledge in existence at the time they are produced is sufficient to represent the whole truth.

At the time when Hill produced his theory, and when Douglas, Haldane and Haldane (9) published their expansion of it, the authors in question had at their disposal a knowledge of colloid chemistry which was denied to Hüfner and to Bohr.

Hill's theory regards the hæmoglobin molecule which contains one atom of iron and which has a molecular weight of about 17,000, as being the unit, which may be represented by the symbol Hb. These units he regarded as capable of combining into aggregates. Any particular aggregate, which now becomes a molecule, was denoted as $(Hb)_m$.

In a solution of hæmoglobin—I use the word "solution" in its strict sense—Hill supposed that there were aggregates of all sorts of sizes, so that m had all sorts of values but the average value of m was n. On this point Hill's theory has been much misunderstood. When he used the symbol $(Hb)_n$ he did not conceive that each aggregate consisted of n molecular units but that n was the average value of m, where m represented the number of units in each aggregate, the values of m in any particular solution being very various. Granting the above assumption, and another, namely, that all the hæmoglobin aggregates are either oxyhæmoglobin or reduced hæmoglobin, the equation for the formation of oxyhæmoglobin would be as follows:

$$Hb_n + nO_2 \rightleftarrows Hb_nO_{2n}.$$

A word concerning the second assumption. It means that intermediate substances between reduced hæmoglobin and oxyhæmoglobin cannot exist in a stable condition. Consider a case, for instance, of a molecule in which $m = 2$. One might suppose, following the usual chemical analogies, that the oxygen might be added in two stages:

(1) $Hb_2 + O_2 = Hb_2O_2$.
(2) $Hb_2O_2 + O_2 = Hb_2O_4$.

Hill's assumption did not preclude such a mode of formation. It stipulated, however, that should two molecules of Hb_2O_2 exist they should at once break up thus:

$$2Hb_2O_2 = Hb_2 + Hb_2O_4.$$

On the reasoning of chemical analogies, the assumption was never quite an easy one. So far as the facts are concerned, no substance intermediate between reduced hæmoglobin and oxyhæmoglobin is known to exist.

The smallest value which m can have is unity, and the simplest hæmoglobin solution of which one can conceive on Hill's theory is one in which there was no aggregation and in which, therefore, $m = 1$. In that case the equation would be

$$Hb + O_2 \rightleftarrows HbO_2,$$

as in Hüfner's theory. Hüfner's theory is therefore included in and is the simplest case of Hill's theory. The corresponding curve is, as we have seen, a rectangular hyperbola.

The above equation, expressed in dynamical terms, would be

$$K \, [Hb] \, [O_2] = [HbO_2];$$

replacing $[O_2]$ by $\frac{x\alpha}{760}$, where x is the pressure of oxygen, and α the solubility, calling HbO_2 the percentage saturation y and Hb $100 - y$, and further remembering that α and 760 are constants and therefore may be included in K, the above equation becomes

$$K \, (100 - y) \, (x) = y,$$

which may be written

$$\frac{y}{100} = \frac{Kx}{1 + Kx}.$$

That is if $m = 1$, but if $m = 2$ the equation would become

$$\frac{y}{100} = \frac{Kx^2}{1 + Kx^2},$$

or if $m = n$, Hill's well-known equation is obtained:

$$\frac{y}{100} = \frac{Kx^n}{1 + Kx^n}.$$

Among its merits is the fact that it contains but two variables, K and n. In spite of this fact the equation, by suitable modifications of these, can be made to yield curves which agree pretty closely to those which have been determined experimentally. The idea of aggregation is supported by the important work of Rona and Yippö [13].

The theory, however, only purports to be a first approximation, because any curve drawn from the equation assumes that when the oxygen pressure is varied the only effect on the hæmoglobin is to vary the quantity of oxygen with which the hæmoglobin unites. This is known now not to be so. To take a single factor: when the oxygen pressure is reduced and a portion of the hæmoglobin changed from oxyhæmoglobin to reduced hæmoglobin, the hydrogen-ion concentration of the fluid is altered. This alteration in itself influences the shape of the curve. If the hæmoglobin were kept at constant hydrogen-ion concentration (the condition to which Hill's equation should rightly be applied) the curve would be somewhat more inflected than the curve determined in the ordinary way and which has the same pressure at 50 per cent. saturation. Such a curve might easily obey Hill's equation with a variation in the value of n, but the matter has not been put to any exhaustive test.

Since Hill's theory was propounded the atmosphere surrounding hæmoglobin has changed. Adair[10] and Svedberg[11] have independently arrived at the conclusion that the molecular weight of hæmoglobin is at its simplest $(16,700)_4$, i.e. $n = 4$, and in the case of the latter research it was clear that 4 is not an average figure but is the actual value for each molecule. Therefore, if Hill's theory was held now, it would resolve itself into a statement that the basic equation was

$$\frac{y}{100} = \frac{Kx^4}{1 + Kx^4}.$$

In so far as this equation does not fit actual curves (and it fits no actual curve determined experimentally) some reason must be shown for the introduction of a correction. This point has been discussed by Adair and will be considered as part of his theory.

Douglas, Haldane and Haldane's[9] *theory* is based on Hill's idea of aggregation, but it introduces another complication, namely, that each time the hæmoglobin aggregate unites with oxygen it breaks up into simple molecules and each of these, having taken up its load of oxygen, re-aggregates.

Moreover, the oxyhæmoglobin and the reduced hæmoglobin do not aggregate to the same extent. The tendency of the reduced hæmoglobin to aggregate is greater than that of the oxyhæmoglobin. There are therefore several reactions taking place at the same time and all obeying the law of mass action:

$$Hb + Hb \rightleftarrows Hb_2,$$
$$Hb_2 + Hb \rightleftarrows Hb_3,$$
$$Hb_3 + Hb \rightleftarrows Hb_4, \text{ etc.};$$

also

$$HbO_2 + HbO_2 \rightleftarrows Hb_2O_4,$$
$$HbO_2 + Hb_2O_4 \rightleftarrows Hb_3O_6,$$
$$HbO_2 + Hb_3O_6 \rightleftarrows Hb_4O_8, \text{ etc.};$$

as well as the reaction of hæmoglobin with oxygen, which can only take place as the result of the disruption of these units.

Precisely analogous is the reaction of hæmoglobin with carbon monoxide; the reduced hæmoglobin and the carboxyhæmoglobin respectively aggregate—the latter more readily than the former.

Lastly, if oxygen and carbon monoxide are both present a series of compounds is formed, which are mixed aggregates of the oxy- and carboxyhæmoglobin:

$$HbO_2 + HbCO \rightleftarrows Hb_2 (O_2) (CO), \text{ etc.}$$

About the aggregates of the last type it must be admitted that they have never been isolated and further, as far as is known at present, their formation does not affect the spectrum. It has never been claimed that an actual mixture of 50 per cent. oxyhæmoglobin and 50 per cent. carboxyhæmoglobin is spectroscopically different from an optical mixture of the two substances—the former would consist largely of the mixed aggregates from which the latter would be free.

The equation, which expresses the shape of the dissociation curve on the theory under consideration, is

$$x = \frac{Ky[1 + b(1 - y)]^*}{(1 - y)(1 + ay)}.$$

x in the above equation is the oxygen pressure expressed in hundredths of an atmosphere, y is the fraction of the total hæmoglobin (taken as unity) which is oxyhæmoglobin, K is the equilibrium constant, whilst a and b are constants referring to the degree of aggregation of the oxy- and reduced hæmoglobin respectively. Thus, "the values $a = 2$, $b = 8$ mean that in fully oxidised hæmoglobin $\frac{2}{3}$ of the oxy-hæmoglobin is aggregated and $\frac{1}{3}$ free, and in completely reduced blood $\frac{8}{9}$ of the reduced hæmoglobin is aggregated and $\frac{1}{9}$ free."

The theory would probably not be regarded by the authors now as being in nearly as strong a position as when it was published, for it implies that the osmotic pressure of a solution of oxyhæmoglobin is greater than one of reduced hæmoglobin, which Adair has shown by experiment not to be the case. Both have a molecular weight of 68,000.

L. J. Henderson's theory. Henderson (12), in criticising Hill's theory, took exception to the very large changes in the value of K, pointing out the want of analogy for, say, hundredfold variations in the equilibrium constant of a reaction, wrought by such means as altera-tions in hydrogen-ion concentration (I pass over the implication that $Hb_4 + 4O_2 = Hb_4O_8$ is the same reaction as $Hb + O_2 = HbO_2$). Henderson therefore put forward a theory in which the value of the equilibrium constant does not suffer more than a twentyfold

* In the original paper the dividend is given as $Ky[1 - b(1 - y)]$—a misprint in the sign.

variation—a conception which appears to be true of dilute solutions according to the kinetic evidence. There is no corresponding kinetic evidence with regard to strong solutions.

Henderson started from the fact that if the solution be acidified the hæmoglobin unites less readily with oxygen, while if the solution be rendered more alkaline the hæmoglobin unites more readily with oxygen. Now the addition of oxygen to reduced hæmoglobin makes the solution more acid, and at first sight one might therefore expect the hæmoglobin to lose its grip of its oxygen but, according to Henderson, there is a difference between increasing the hydrogen-ion concentration of a hæmoglobin solution by the addition of acid and increasing it by the addition of oxygen. The former makes the hæmoglobin solution unite with less base, the latter makes the hæmoglobin unite with more base. Therefore—so runs the argument as I understand it— the addition of oxygen to hæmoglobin, while it renders the solution more acid, makes the hæmoglobin behave in the same way as would the addition of alkali to the solution: that is, it causes the hæmo-globin to unite more readily with oxygen and thus changes what would have been a hyperbolic into an inflected curve.

I think Henderson's theory really amounts to this:

(a) That in any hæmoglobin solution there exist the following substances which I shall for the moment call by names that will indicate their compositions:

(1) Hæmoglobinic acid.
(2) Sodium hæmoglobinate.
(3) Oxyhæmoglobinic acid.
(4) Sodium oxyhæmoglobinate.

(b) That therefore from the point of view of the oxygen there are two equilibria:

(1) $H.Hb + O_2 \rightleftarrows H.HbO_2$.
(2) $Na.Hb + O_2 \rightleftarrows Na.HbO_2$.

(c) That the quantity of sodium hæmoglobinate increases gradually as the hæmoglobin acquires oxygen.

(d) That the sodium hæmoglobinate system has a much stronger affinity for oxygen than the hæmoglobinic acid system. The final dissociation curve is a composite of the dissociation curves of the two systems.

This theory has much that is attractive. It is capable of being elaborated by making various assumptions, and I have little doubt that it could be put into such a form by mathematicians as to make it fit either the known curves or others. I tried to draw the curves, making some rather simple assumptions, but without any success. Starting from the assumption of a hyperbola for each reaction I did not get an S-shaped curve, but a curve, the tangent to any part of which cut the x axis to the left of the origin.

It would appear, as Adair has pointed out, that the theory is to some extent capable of experimental verification. If the hæmoglobin solution is in any case very alkaline, even when reduced, the pigment would be present mostly in the form of sodium hæmoglobinate; if, on the other hand, there is no base in the solution, the sodium component would be absent. In either case a curve of hyperbolic nature should be found, whilst the double inflection would be most prominent near the isoelectric point. The evidence on this point clearly needs strengthening.

Some curves worked out by Adair, Bock and myself and published in the *Harvey Lectures*, 1921–1922, p. 156, are just of the type which would fit in with Henderson's theory, but the subsequent and more exhaustive researches of Adair have yielded curves which, when corrected for progressive difference of hydrogen-ion concentration of the fluid as the material becomes oxidised, show almost no change in inflection from one hydrogen-ion concentration to another.

Adair's theory (14). According to Hill's theory the value of n as calculated from the dissociation curve of a solution of hæmoglobin should be the same as that actually found with an osmometer. It was to test this point that Adair took up the measurement of the osmotic pressure of hæmoglobin. In a former chapter the matter has been dealt with in detail. Here it need only be said that in dilute solutions at the isoelectric point Adair finds the osmotic pressure to correspond to a molecular weight of 68,000, or thereabouts, and thus to a molecule which corresponds to four units, in short, to Hb_4. It will be gathered from what has already been said that this determination cuts right across all preconceived ideas of the constitution of hæmoglobin. Clearly on the lines of Hill's equation, if n equalled 4 the curve of pure hæmoglobin would be even more inflected than that of blood, whilst the work which had been done on the subject indicated that in such a condition the dissociation curve would be a rectangular hyperbola. To that point we will return. In the meantime, passing from dilute solutions, by which is meant solutions of, say, 1 per cent. to 0·1 per cent., to solutions of the same order of concentration as blood, say, 15 per cent., Adair finds an apparent osmotic pressure corresponding to a value for n of about 2·5. His view is, however, not that the hæmoglobin becomes less aggregated as it becomes more concentrated, but that the molecules are so close together as to interfere with one another's freedom, and also with one another's power of receiving their rightful number of oxygen impacts. Thus, starting with the assumption that the fundamental equation is

$$Hb_4 + 4O_2 = Hb_4O_8,$$

a correction has to be introduced in order to express the degree to which each molecule screens its fellow from oxygen. The lines along which Adair argues are those which have already been applied to sugar solutions. It is known that whereas a dilute sugar solution obeys the law

$$PV = RT,$$

where P is the osmotic pressure, V is the volume in litres of solution per gram molecule, R is the gas constant and T the absolute temperature, a strong solution behaves as though it had a lower pressure than the number of molecules would indicate, and a correction b has to be subtracted from the volume so that the form of the equation for a strong solution of hæmoglobin would be

$$P(V - b) = RT.$$

For hæmoglobin $b = 162$ litres, according to Adair, and V is the volume in litres which contains 67,000 grams of hæmoglobin.

Take for instance a 14 per cent. solution of hæmoglobin; 67,000 grams of hæmoglobin would occupy 480 litres. So the equation would stand

$$P(480 - 162) = RT.$$

P, therefore, would be higher than might be expected, that is to say, the solution would behave as though more molecules were present, i.e. as though the hæmoglobin were in a less state of aggregation.

It is interesting to apply this conception as Adair did to Hill's equation, for Hill was very clear that n in his equation did not mean the actual state of aggregation, but such state of aggregation as might be deduced from the osmotic pressure. Therefore, in this case, n would equal not 4, but something under 3, and that value would give a curve which, when corrected for hydrogen-ion concentration, would be very near to that actually found for blood.

Hill's equation would stand

$$Kx^3 = \frac{y\,(1 + \cdot12y)}{1 - y}.$$

This equation corresponds well with the curve for blood.

But there are difficulties:

The first is that though 100 grams of blood contain about 14 grams of hæmoglobin, it cannot be said to be a 14 per cent. solution of hæmoglobin. The corpuscle is about a 30 per cent. solution. The calculation on that basis becomes much more difficult to accept.

The second is that, according to the assumptions which we have made, the dissociation curve of a dilute solution should be more inflected than that of a strong solution. And the experimental evidence is against that view.

The bulk of evidence still seems to support the idea that the dissociation curve of hæmoglobin reduced to its simplest terms is a rectangular hyperbola. The evidence for this is:

(1) The work of Barcroft and Roberts[15], which gave a curve approximating to that shape.

(2) The work of Hartridge and Roughton[16] which, at every point at which the matter could be tested, indicated that in dilute solutions the reaction between hæmoglobin and oxygen was a bimolecular one.

(3) That Hecht and Morgan[17] did on three occasions obtain a very perfect rectangular hyperbola, while the curves which they obtained on other occasions were intermediate in inflection between that of blood and the hyperbola.

Now the question arises: Can these difficulties be cleared away? Is the reaction

$$Hb_4 + 4O_2 \rightleftharpoons Hb_4O_8$$

capable of being represented graphically by a rectangular hyperbola? The answer is in the affirmative, but certain assumptions must be made which may be integrated in the statement that the reaction must be regarded as four bimolecular reactions taking place independently, thus:

$$Hb_4 \quad + O_2 \rightleftharpoons Hb_4O_2$$
$$Hb_4O_2 + O_2 \rightleftharpoons Hb_4O_4$$
$$Hb_4O_4 + O_2 \rightleftharpoons Hb_4O_6$$
$$Hb_4O_6 + O_2 \rightleftharpoons Hb_4O_8.$$

If the reaction were of this character, and the molecule large enough to allow of the supposition that each molecule of combined oxygen was quite uninfluenced by the others, then one might expect a rectangular hyperbola as the dissociation curve.

Now the hypothesis that the molecules of iron are so far from one another that their activities can be regarded as independent is not unreasonable, and the existence of intermediate oxides, Hb_4O_2, Hb_4O_4 and Hb_4O_6, is what might be expected on chemical analogies. So far, so good. The reader may ask with reason, Where is the difficulty? Firstly, there is the fact that these intermediate oxides have never been observed either spectroscopically or otherwise. If you present hæmoglobin with, say, one-quarter the amount of oxygen necessary for its saturation, there is no evidence of Hb_4O_2. Now this difficulty might conceivably be met by the assumption that the oxides are unstable. That explanation cannot be accepted; in theory it is the same thing as saying that they do not exist, and is in fact the assumption made by Hill as the basis of his equation, which would be

$$\frac{y}{100} = \frac{Kx^4}{1 + Kx^4}.$$

Secondly, it makes no provision for the curve ever being other than a hyperbola.

The best appreciation of the situation which can be given at present seems to be the following:

1. Fundamentally we must start with weak solutions.
2. The molecular weight of hæmoglobin in such is 67,000, or $(16,700)_4$.
3. The reaction with oxygen is

$$Hb_4 + 4O_2 = Hb_4O_8.$$

4. The dissociation curve of the reaction with O_2 or CO in weak solutions is very far from being expressed by the equation

$$\frac{y}{100} = \frac{Kx^4}{1 + Kx^4}.$$

5. The dissociation curve is very near to being

$$\frac{y}{100} = \frac{Kx}{1 + Kx}.$$

6. The facts contained in paragraphs 1–5 (above) can be reconciled by assuming the existence of intermediate oxides, which exist for a finite time, but which have never been seen.

7. They leave unexplained the more familiar dissociation curve of blood

$$\frac{y}{100} = \frac{Kx^{2\cdot5}}{1 + Kx^{2\cdot5}}.$$

REFERENCES

(1) OSTWALD, WOLFGANG. *Biochem. Ctrlb.* p. 386. 1908.
(2) BROWN, W. E. L. *Nature*, CXI. 881. 1923.
(3) ADAM, K. N. *Nature*. CXI. 496. 1923.
(4) CONANT AND SCOTT. *Journ. Biol. Chem.* LXVIII. 107. 1926.
(5) HÜFNER. *Arch. f. Anat. u. Physiol.* Suppl. 187. 1901.
(6) BOHR, CHRISTIAN. *Zentralb. f. Physiol.* XVII. 682. 1903.
(7) HILL, A. V. *Journ. Physiol.* XL. *Physiol. Soc. Proc.* iv. 1910. *Biochem. Journ.* VII. 471. 1913. *Journ. Biol. Chem.* LI. 395. 1922.
(8) BARCROFT, J. *Biochem. Journ.* VII. 482. 1913.
(9) DOUGLAS, C. G., HALDANE, J. B. S. AND HALDANE, J. S. *Journ. Physiol.* XLIV. 275. 1912.
(10) ADAIR. *Proc. Roy. Soc.* A. CVIII. 628. 1925.
(11) SVEDBERG. *Journ. Amer. Chem. Soc.* XLVIII. 430. 1926.
(12) HENDERSON, L. J. *Journ. Biol. Chem.* XLI. 416. 1920.
(13) RONA AND YIPPÖ. *Biochem. Zeitsch.* LXXVI. 187. 1916.
(14) ADAIR. *Journ. Biol. Chem.* LXIII. 533. 1925.
(15) BARCROFT AND ROBERTS. *Journ. Physiol.* XXXIX. 143. 1909.
(16) HARTRIDGE AND ROUGHTON. *Proc. Roy. Soc.* A. CVII. 654. 1925.
(17) HECHT AND MORGAN. In press.

CHAPTER XIII

THE KINETICS OF OXYHÆMOGLOBIN
IN DILUTE SOLUTIONS

Now to return to theoretical considerations. At the commencement of the previous chapter we showed that one theory at least of the union of oxygen with hæmoglobin required that the equilibrium curve should be a rectangular hyperbola. The theory was that a simple reaction took place between one molecule of oxygen and one molecule

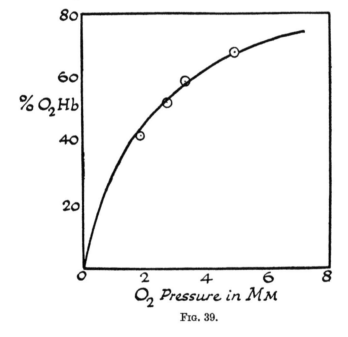

FIG. 39.

of reduced hæmoglobin, following the laws of mass action. This is not the only theory which might lead to a hyperbolic equilibrium curve—the point is that this theory can lead to no other. The argument which led us up to our conclusion assumed that the equilibrium constant of the reaction K was the ratio of two velocity constants, k' and k; the former represented the rate at which oxyhæmoglobin broke down into oxygen and hæmoglobin, the latter the rate in the same units at which oxygen and hæmoglobin united to form oxy-hæmoglobin.

Clearly we should be putting our theory to a very rigorous test by determining k' and k independently and then ascertaining whether their ratio corresponded to the equilibrium constant of the hyperbola as determined. This latter may be obtained from Fig. 39 (1).

Hill and I, and later Oinuma, made some tentative efforts in this direction by bubbling oxygen through hæmoglobin solutions and observing the rate at which the solution became oxidised, and conversely bubbling nitrogen through solutions of oxyhæmoglobin and observing the period necessary for reduction (2), (3). It became evident very early that, important as these results undoubtedly are from another standpoint, we were observing something fundamentally different from the velocity constants of the reactions in question. Our curves really indicated the rates at which the solution acquired or lost oxygen, as will be shown in Chapter XVI.

Data obtained in this way reflect, to some extent, the properties of the equilibrium curves of the reactions involved. They do not, however, yield any information concerning the time required for the actual chemical process of union or disintegration of the hæmoglobin to take place.

These latter involve intervals of time which are infinitesimal in relation to those necessary for the oxygen to diffuse into the solution when bubbled through it at a convenient rate.

The independent measurement of k and k' for the reactions

$$Hb + O_2 \longrightarrow HbO_2$$
$$HbO_2 \longrightarrow Hb + O_2$$

has been undertaken and brought to a triumphant conclusion by Hartridge and Roughton. Their researches are notable in physiology as being the first in which the velocity constants of any so simple a reaction in the body have been measured, and in chemistry as being the first in which a reaction of such rapidity has been made to yield its secret.

Of the two reactions, the acquisition of hæmoglobin by oxygen is the more rapid and therefore the more difficult to measure. The time interval which is involved in the measurement is expressed in thousandths of a second.

To give a detailed account of the complete fabric of this research is beyond the scope of a chapter in the present book. I must satisfy myself—but I hope not the reader—by setting forth the principles which underlie it. The reader can, and I hope will, refer to Hartridge and Roughton's original papers for more detailed knowledge[4].

Two solutions, I and II, the former of reduced hæmoglobin, the latter of oxygenated water, are prepared. Solution I contains hæmoglobin in about one-fortieth of the concentration in which it is present in blood. Solution II contains the minimal quantity of oxygen necessary for the reaction, thus making it as slow as possible. These solutions are driven along rubber tubing and meet in a special apparatus. This apparatus consists of a glass tube, at one end of which—that at which they enter—there is a contrivance for mixing the fluids. The fluids there are brought instantly into intimate contact after which they traverse a glass tube. If the flow along the tube is sufficiently rapid, about 600 cm. per second, it is possible to detect a change of colour in the first few centimetres. At first the fluid is appreciably "venous" in colour: it rapidly becomes "arterial." It is possible to examine, spectroscopically, the fluid at various fixed points in this zone of changing colour and thus to determine the relative quantities of oxy- and reduced hæmoglobin at each station. Knowing the velocity at which the fluid is running, the rate at which it changes from being a mixture of reduced hæmoglobin and oxygen to being a compound of the two can be calculated.

It is necessary to be certain that the time thus measured is actually taken up by the act of chemical combination, and not merely by the complete mixing of the oxygen solution with that of the hæmo- globin. Hartridge and Roughton[4] made sure of their ground in this respect in the following way. The solutions I and II were replaced by an alkaline solution which contained phenol-phthalein and an acid solution respectively. The strengths of acid and alkali were such that the mixed fluid would be just acid and therefore the indicator would be bleached. Before the red colour could disappear completely three things then must have happened: (1) the complete mixture of the solutions, (2) the chemical action between the alkali and the acid, (3) the reaction between the excess of acid (very dilute) and the phenol-phthalein. Clearly the time which these three processes jointly would require would exceed that occupied by the first—the mere mixing. Yet the mixing was so rapid and so intimate that no red colour could be detected beyond the first few millimetres of the tube.

The second experimental precaution to which I shall allude is one which ensures that at any particular spot the fluid over the whole

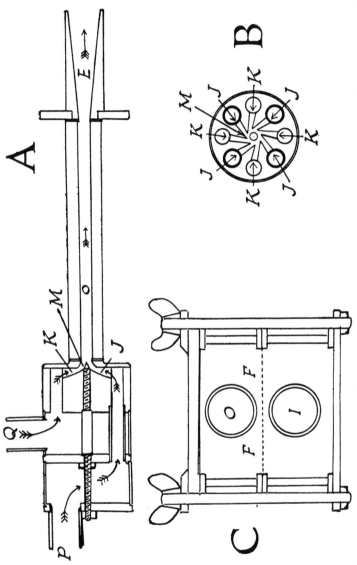

FIG. 40, A. Diagrammatic longitudinal section of the mixing apparatus principally used for the work recorded in this chapter. The reduced hæmoglobin and the oxygenated water enter respectively through the pipes P and Q. They are then forced through the four jets J and the four jets K respectively, and enter the mixing chamber M, from which they pass immediately into the observation tube O, to flow finally out at the exit E.

B. Arrangement of the jets J and K with regard to the mixing chamber.

C. Arrangement of the two filter boxes through which the fluids passed on their way from the bottles to the apparatus. Fluids enter at I, pass through the copper or brass gauge F, and leave again at O.

The thumb nuts enable the apparatus to be readily taken to pieces for cleaning and to be assembled again afterwards.

cross-section of the glass tube is of uniform composition. It would not be unnatural to assume a stream line flow, with the possibility that the fluid in the core was flowing more rapidly and was of different composition to the layers situate in close contact to the glass.

Some idea was formed of the nature of the flow by forcing two fluids through the apparatus which by nature did not mix—coloured water and paraffin. Experiments of this character indicated a rotary motion in the outer layers of the fluid, and indeed, bubbles visible in the fluid suggested the question whether a core in the axis was not moving towards the mixing chamber instead of away from it.

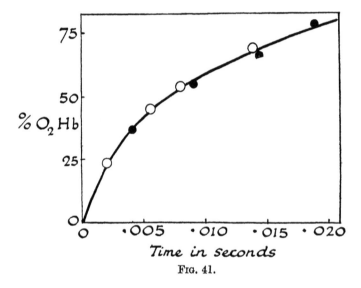

Fig. 41.

"Three independent tests were applied in order to answer this question: (1) to cause alternately colourless and coloured fluid to pass down the observation tube, (2) to compare spectroscopic readings taken through the centre of the tube, which would therefore include the core, with those taken through the periphery of the tube, which would not include the core, (3) to compare spectroscopic readings obtained on one and the same reaction at slow and fast speeds....Our conclusion is that all parts of the fluid travel with the same velocity down the tube."

The results of some tests in which the fluids passed at very different rates along the observation tube are shown in Fig. 41: "the shaded circles representing readings obtained with a slow linear flow (96 cm. per sec.) and the blank circles representing readings obtained with a fast rate of linear flow (333 cm. per sec.). The two reacting solutions were in each of the experiments identical."

To pass now from the method to the results which it achieved; they are of course subject to a large percentage error, considerably over 20 per cent.

The results of an experiment at pH 7·7 and temperature 17·5 are as follows:

The times are measured from the earliest obtainable reading. It will be noted that the time taken to reach half-completion is less than one seven-hundredth of a second.

The value of k' for the interval $t = 0$—0·00184 sec. is 106, and for the interval $t = 0·00184$—0·00370 sec. is 157; the mean being 132.

Our interest in the above experiment lies in the fact that the velocity constant in the later portion of the reaction is not less than in the earlier portion.

A second experiment, carried out on similar lines, gave results which varied from 120 to 130. Taking the mean of observations made under those particular conditions of temperature and hydrogen-ion concentration the value for k' averages out at 128 plus or minus over 10 per cent.

Though particular pains were taken in the regulation of the hydrogen-ion concentration by means of a buffer and in the observation of the temperature, it is noteworthy that the velocity of the reaction

$$Hb + O_2 \longrightarrow HbO_2$$

is almost independent of changes in either of the factors mentioned.

It has been observed above that the velocity constant of the reaction is the same over the whole of its course. This does not mean that the rate of formation of oxyhæmoglobin is the same at the end of the reaction as at the commencement, and indeed Fig. 41 shows it to be otherwise. Towards the end of the reaction less oxyhæmoglobin is being formed in a given interval of time than at the commencement. There are two reasons for this. The first is that the formation of oxyhæmoglobin at any moment is proportional to the products of the concentrations of reduced hæmoglobin and oxygen, which are ever becoming diminishing quantities. The second is that as oxyhæmoglobin is present in increasing amounts it tends more and more to break up and set the reaction in the opposite direction. The measurement would in theory be much easier if the oxyhæmoglobin immediately on formation were removed from the system. It has not been found possible to do this, and therefore the effect of the accumulating oxyhæmoglobin must be allowed for by calculation. This allowance can be made if the velocity constant for the reaction,

$$HbO_2 \rightarrow Hb + O_2,$$

be known.

The question may be asked with reason: Does not just the same argument apply to the reaction,

$$HbO_2 \rightarrow Hb + O_2,$$

as to the oxidation? Is it possible to find the velocity constant for the reduction of hæmoglobin without a knowledge of that for the oxidation? And indeed the argument would appear to have great force inasmuch as the velocity constant for the oxidation is much greater than for the reduction. The answer is that Hartridge and Roughton have broken this vicious circle in the following way[5]. They have succeeded, in the case of the reduction, in removing the oxygen from the sphere of action as quickly as it is formed; this they achieved by the presence in the system of the reducing agent, sodium hydrosulphite—$Na_2S_2O_4$.

Let us turn to the consideration of Hartridge and Roughton's experiments for the measurement of the velocity constant for the reaction

$$HbO_2 \rightarrow Hb + O_2.$$

The apparatus was essentially the same in nature as that which we have already described, but inasmuch as the reaction is slower, the whole apparatus does not require to be so powerful. A slower current along the observation tube suffices, powerful pumps for the propulsion of the fluids are unnecessary, and the pressures inside the apparatus are not so great but that it can be assembled from ordinary laboratory materials. The reacting fluids led into the observation tube were, fluid I, a solution of oxyhæmoglobin, which necessarily contained dissolved oxygen and which was buffered to the required hydrogen-ion concentration; fluid II, a solution of hydrosulphite, which in the nature of the case was free from dissolved oxygen—any such would at once be taken up by the hydrosulphite.

When the fluids met, the following sequence of events took place. Firstly, the hydrosulphite ate up the oxygen in solution. Secondly, when the oxygen pressure in the fluid was reduced to a few millimetres (the temperature being 15·5° C.) the oxyhæmoglobin commenced to yield its oxygen, which for a moment went into physical solution. Thirdly, this oxygen was immediately laid hold upon by the hydrosulphite. These three processes ran their courses until the whole of the oxyhæmoglobin was reduced.

It is necessary to be very clear that the events which took place were precisely those which we have described; the other obvious possibility being that the oxyhæmoglobin was reduced directly by the hydrosulphite by a process of double decomposition. The authors investigated this matter in great detail and seem to have left no reasonable doubt that their view is correct.

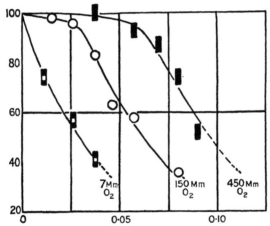

FIG. 42. Abscissa = time in seconds. Ordinate = Percentage oxyhæmoglobin observations obtained when oxygen pressure in solution was initially
    (i)   7 mm. Hg, represented by striped rectangles;
    (ii) 150 mm. Hg,   ,,   circles;
    (iii) 450 mm. Hg,   ,,   black rectangles.
Temperature = 15·5° C.

Here we have a reaction which, of course, gradually becomes slower in the sense that the amount of oxyhæmoglobin which breaks down in any small moment of time is proportional to the remaining, though ever decreasing, concentration of oxyhæmoglobin in the solution. This being so the logarithm of the quantity of oxyhæmoglobin present, when plotted against the time which has elapsed since the commencement of the experiment, should produce a straight line.

Figures 42, 43 and 44 illustrate the points which have been mentioned. Fig. 42 shows the course of three experiments, in each the concentration of oxyhæmoglobin (i.e. the percentage saturation from 100 per cent. downwards) is plotted against the time which has elapsed since the fluids came together. The curves are marked respectively 7 mm. O_2, 150 mm. O_2 and 450 mm. O_2. These figures signify the partial pressures of, and are therefore measures of, the oxygen present physically dissolved in solution I. It is clear that the greater the quantity of oxygen which is thus *dissolved*, the longer will the hydrosulphite take in ridding the mixture completely of it, and therefore the longer the time which will elapse before the reduction of the hæmoglobin commences. Herein lies the significance of the fact that the graph marked 7 mm. O_2 descends abruptly from the origin: any decrease in the dissolved oxygen below 7 mm. entails an appreciable reduction of the hæmoglobin. The two remaining graphs descend but little from the 100 per cent. level for a time—longer in the case of the solution which has the higher concentration of free oxygen. It is to be noted that the three graphs, once they do take a definitely downward course, are parallel to one another, showing that the reaction

$$HbO_2 \longrightarrow Hb + O_2$$

proceeds at the same rate in each case.

As has been indicated the curves gradually tend to become less steep, because the amount of oxyhæmoglobin broken up in a given moment of time depends upon the amount of oxyhæmoglobin which is left unbroken in the solution at that time. If, however, this law is rigidly fulfilled—and it is simply the law of mass action adapted to this particular case—the logarithm of the concentration of oxyhæmoglobin, when plotted against the time through which the reaction has run, should give a straight line. This is another way of saying that the velocity constant of the reaction is the same from start to finish, and of saying that if the same concentration of oxyhæmoglobin were present in each case, the time necessary for a certain small proportion of it to be broken up would be the same irrespective of the amount of reduced hæmoglobin with which it were mixed, i.e. irrespective of the percentage saturation.

Fig. 43 shows that Hartridge and Roughton's determinations, when plotted in the way indicated above, fall on a straight line with exactitude of a remarkable order considering the difficulties under which they were made.

On page 139 an experiment was cited in which the velocity constant for the reaction

$$Hb + O_2 \longrightarrow HbO_2$$

was given as being represented by the figure 132. A determination of the velocity constant of the opposite phase, viz.

$$HbO_2 \longrightarrow Hb + \cdot O_2,$$

was made on the same hæmoglobin solution and yielded the figure 17·5.

The ratio of these two velocity constants,

$$\frac{132}{17\cdot5} = 7\cdot5,$$

should give the equilibrium constant of the reaction

$$HbO_2 \rightleftarrows H_2b + O_2$$

indirectly, and this, as was pointed out at the commencement of the chapter, should agree with the equilibrium constant as obtained from

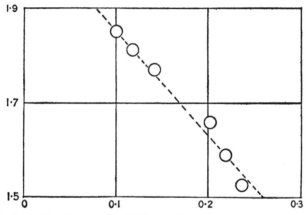

FIG. 43. Abscissa = time in seconds. Ordinate = log. of percentage of oxyhæmoglobin.

Fig. 39, for it was determined from the same solution. That equilibrium constant, in the units used above, worked out to 9·75. Considering the magnitude of the errors involved this degree of agreement is highly satisfactory.

Stress has been laid upon the fact that all the determinations necessary for the above comparison were carried out on the same solution of hæmoglobin. For this there are several reasons, two of which may now be stated; the reduction phase,

$$HbO_2 \longrightarrow Hb + O_2,$$

unlike the oxidation phase, is very sensitive to the conditions under which it takes place, notably, the hydrogen-ion concentration and the temperature.

Some more detailed information may be given on these relationships before the chapter closes.

Fig. 44 is similar to Fig. 43, but instead of showing the relation of the logarithm of the percentage saturation of oxyhæmoglobin to the time in the case of a single solution of hæmoglobin, it depicts that relation for a number of such solutions, the hydrogen-ion concentrations of which differ. The figure attached to each line indicates the pH of the solution to which the line refers. As the alkalinity increases so the rate of reduction becomes slower, but not uniformly so; evidently between pH 6·9 and 7·7 a given change in reaction has

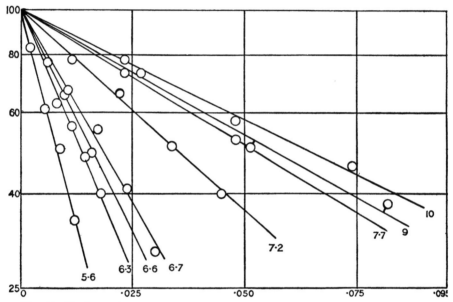

Fig. 44. Abscissa = time in seconds. Ordinate = oxyhæmoglobin percentage; numerals on left of ordinate axis indicate corresponding value of oxyhæmoglobin percentage.

a much greater effect upon the slope of the line than in the more acid and more alkaline regions. Indeed, above pH 8 increased alkalinity has but little effect on the velocity constant, and the same is probably true, though the experimental evidence is more meagre, below pH 5. It is only in the region of the isoelectric point that hydrogen-ion concentration greatly influences the rate at which hæmoglobin breaks up. The hydrogen-ion concentration of the blood is, however, about 7·4–7·6 and is therefore that at which the velocity constant of the reduction phase is most sensitive to temperature. The relation between the velocity constant for the reaction

$$HbO_2 \longrightarrow Hb + O_2$$

and the exponent of the hydrogen-ion concentration is shown in Fig. 45.

The effect of temperature on the rate of the reaction

$$HbO_2 \longrightarrow Hb + O_2$$

is also in strong contrast to its effect—or lack of effect—on the rate of the reaction

$$Hb + O_2 \longrightarrow HbO_2.$$

Hartridge and Roughton made a series of measurements, both on acid and alkaline solutions, and found that the velocity constant in each case had the high temperature coefficient, 3·8. In the case of the acid solution ($pH = 5\cdot6$) it was practicable to get measurements only between 3° and 14° C., but in the case of the alkaline solution

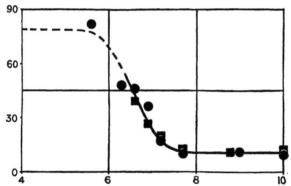

FIG. 45. Abscissa $= pH$ of solution. Ordinate $=$ value of reduction velocity constant. Squares represent results obtained in experiment on one sample of blood. Circles represent results obtained in experiment on another sample of blood.

($pH = 9$), in which the reaction goes more slowly, data were obtainable up to 28° C. In both cases the observations which were made inspire a good deal of confidence, since they fall into line with the demands of Arrhenius' equation

$$\log \frac{K_1}{K_2} = \frac{\mu}{R}\left(\frac{1}{T_2} - \frac{1}{T_1}\right),$$

according to which the logarithm of the velocity constant should vary directly with the reciprocal of the absolute temperature. How good the agreement is between the observed points and the theory is shown by Fig. 46, B.

Putting together the principal facts about the reduction and oxidation velocities what light may they be expected to shed on the equilibrium curves of oxyhæmoglobin? Three main points emerge.

Firstly, as has already been stated, if all three constants are determined for the same solution, good agreement is found between the ratio of the velocity constants and the equilibrium constant.

Secondly, altered hydrogen-ion concentration, in a certain region, viz. between 5·6 and 9, would be expected to produce a profound change in the equilibrium, because whilst having almost no effect on the oxidation, it greatly facilitates the reduction. The greater the hydrogen-ion concentration, the less oxygen will be taken up at a given pressure.

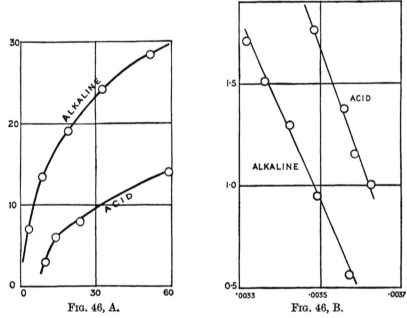

FIG. 46, A.   FIG. 46, B.

A. Abscissa = value of reduction velocity constant. Ordinate = temperature in degrees Centigrade.
B. Abscissa = reciprocal of absolute temperature. Ordinate = logarithm of reduction velocity constant.

Thirdly, a rise of temperature should tend also to reduce the quantity of oxygen taken up at a given oxygen pressure; for the same reason, namely, that whilst the reaction

$$Hb + O_2 \longrightarrow HbO_2$$

has a temperature coefficient of approximately 1, that of the reaction

$$HbO_2 \longrightarrow Hb + O_2$$

is approximately 3·8. The temperature coefficient of the equilibrium constant may therefore be expected to be somewhere about the latter figure.

Variation of concentration of reacting substances. The effect of concentration, as such, has yet to be studied. Hartridge and Roughton had very little choice in the concentration of hæmoglobin and of oxygen which they used; they were tied to the only one which would give their measurements.

The kinetics of oxyhæmoglobin only form one portion of Hartridge and Roughton's work: carboxyhæmoglobin has been studied as well and is discussed in Chapter xv.

Moreover, the spectroscope is not the only method by which they have observed the progress of reactions in their observation tubes. Thermal[5] methods have also been used with success, and these methods are of importance because they render the whole technique available for the exploration of many rapid reactions taking place between colourless reagents.

REFERENCES

(1) HARTRIDGE AND ROUGHTON. *Proc. Roy. Soc.* A. cvii. 643. 1925.
(2) BARCROFT AND HILL. *Journ. Physiol.* xxxix. 411. 1910.
(3) OINUMA. *Journ. Physiol.* xliii. 364. 1911.
(4) HARTRIDGE AND ROUGHTON. *Proc. Roy. Soc.* A. cii. 595. 1923; civ. 376. 1923; civ. 395. 1923; cvii. 654. 1925. *Ibid.* B. xciv. 336 1923.
(5) HARTRIDGE AND ROUGHTON. *Proc. Camb. Phil. Soc.* xxii. 429. 1924.

CHAPTER XIV

THE INTERACTION OF CARBON MONOXIDE
WITH REDUCED HÆMOGLOBIN

The subject of the present chapter is the reaction of carbon monoxide with reduced hæmoglobin, the parallel to that between reduced hæmoglobin and oxygen. It is necessary to be quite clear about the reaction under discussion and not to confuse it with another—that of hæmoglobin with oxygen and carbon monoxide simultaneously. In the language of equations we are dealing in this chapter with

$$Hb + CO \rightleftharpoons HbCO$$

and not with

$$HbO_2 + CO \rightleftharpoons HbCO + O_2,$$

which latter will be discussed in Chapter xv. Until quite recently little attention had been paid to the interaction of carbon monoxide and hæmoglobin in the absence of oxygen.

A controversy ranged at one time about the question whether the number of cubic centimetres of carbon monoxide with which a gram of hæmoglobin could unite was, or was not, exactly the same as the volume of oxygen which attached itself to a gram of the same hæmoglobin. This controversy has faded into the past, and now, oxygen and carbon monoxide are regarded as quantitatively interchangeable; but one never ceases to wonder that two gases which are so different in their properties can play so similar a rôle.

It is not merely that they unite in equal quantities with hæmoglobin. The similarity goes much further. This became evident from the first serious work which was done on the dissociation curve of CO-hæmoglobin, that of Douglas, J. B. S. Haldane and J. S. Haldane[1]. These authors published a series of curves obtained by the carmine method, for the equilibrium of blood with carbon monoxide in the presence of various CO_2-pressures; repeating in effect for carbon monoxide the work which had been done by Bohr, Hasselbalch and Krogh[2] for oxygen.

The comparison is very instructive. In Fig. 47 Douglas, Haldane and Haldane curves for various CO_2-pressures are given, copied directly from their paper. The CO_2-pressures are 0, 19, 41 and 79 mm. respectively. The crosses represent Bohr, Hasselbalch and Krogh's curves for oxyhæmoglobin at approximately the same CO_2-pressures (5, 20, 40 and 80 mm.). The abscissa (on the top of the figure, the oxygen pressure in millimetres) is of course widely different from that for the CO-hæmoglobin, and the scales are so arranged that the point of 50 per cent. saturation on the 80 mm. curve coincides for each series. That is to say, the oxygen pressures throughout for the oxyhæmoglobin curves are 38 : ·156 or 245 times those of the

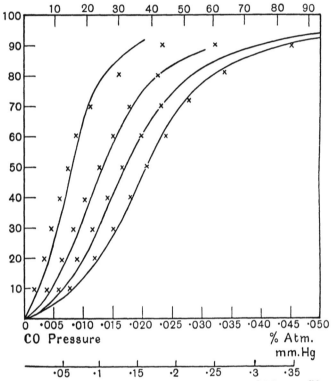

Fig. 47. Equilibrium curves of Hb and CO at 0, 19, 41 and 79 mm. CO_2-pressure respectively. × indicate curves for Hb and O_2 equilibrium drawn with reference to abscissa indicated at the top of the figure.

carbon monoxide for the CO-hæmoglobin curves. The figure 245 we need not discuss here. We shall see later that it depends upon the kind of animal, the temperature, etc. The point is that there is a constant relation over two sets of curves, one for oxy-hæmoglobin and the other for carboxyhæmoglobin, so that in a specified case a number can be given which applies to the whole diagram. In the present case you can say that if a certain pressure of

CO is in equilibrium with a certain percentage of COHb in a certain blood then, under similar circumstances, in another sample of the same blood 245 times that pressure of O_2 will be in equilibrium with the same percentage of oxyhæmoglobin. This statement may be made within limits which are extraordinarily narrow considering that the oxygen curves were done with the old pump and that indeed the curves were extrapolations, i.e. they were contours drawn on what was virtually a surface which represented three variables, the oxygen pressure, the CO_2-pressure and the percentage saturation. While in general the curves given by Douglas, Haldane and Haldane, and those given by Bohr, Hasselbalch and Krogh, are superposable, there is a certain slight systematic difference which might be passed over, but for the fact that it raises a point of theoretical interest. If any pair of corresponding curves be selected, say those at 80 mm. CO_2-pressure, the oxyhæmoglobin curve tends to cross the CO-hæmoglobin curve, being to the left of it at low percentage saturations and to the right of it at high percentage saturations. Now it must be remembered that oxyhæmoglobin is a stronger acid than reduced hæmoglobin and therefore, as the oxygen leaves the corpuscle, the reaction of the inside of the corpuscle becomes more alkaline, which fact would tend to divert the curve to the left. So one may pause a moment to enquire whether the same is true of carbon monoxide. If the carboxyhæmoglobin is not a stronger acid than reduced hæmoglobin we have a qualitative difference between the relationship of oxygen and carbon monoxide to hæmoglobin. This difference, if it existed, might account for the crossing of the curves.

The evidence, however, is in quite the opposite direction. Parsons[3] (using the hydrogen electrode) and the Rockefeller school[4] agree that carbon monoxide produces much the same change of hydrogen-ion concentration in reduced blood as oxygen would do. And on general grounds this is likely to be so, for the change of hydrogen-ion concentration wrought by oxygen or CO on blood is but the counterpart of the change of oxygen (or CO-) content wrought by alteration of the hydrogen-ion concentration. There is reason to believe that the very alterations in O_2-content and CO-content, which correspond so exactly in Fig. 47, are due to changes in hydrogen-ion content and not to specific changes in CO_2. It is likely that saturation, whether with oxygen or CO, will produce the same effect on the hydrogen-ion concentration.

If, therefore, we wish to discover the reason why the curves of

Douglas, Haldane and Haldane(1) tend to cross those of Bohr, Hasselbalch and Krogh (2) we must seek some other explanation. This may perhaps be found in the fact that the latter curves were obtained from the analysis of whole blood, the former from those of dilute blood. (In both cases of course the equilibrium was struck on whole blood.)

Within the last few years much additional interest has been added to the equation

$$CO + Hb \rightleftharpoons HbCO$$

by the work of Hartridge and Roughton(5), for they have taken the reaction out of the region of statics, in which it had hitherto been, and have removed it to the region of kinematics, having extended their brilliant researches to the determination of the velocity constants of the two phases of the reaction respectively.

Firstly, let us consider the reaction

$$CO + Hb \longrightarrow HbCO.$$

Their method was along the same lines as that for the association of oxygen with hæmoglobin. They started with two separate solutions (each free from oxygen), one containing reduced hæmoglobin in a strength of ·2 to ·4 per cent., the other containing distilled water charged with carbon monoxide in solution, into which is introduced some $Na_2S_2O_4$. This latter material, which is a strong reducing agent, ensures the freedom of the system from oxyhæmoglobin whilst itself not affecting the reaction between CO- and reduced hæmoglobin. The two solutions are forced under pressure into a mixing chamber in which they become intimately mixed in a time which is negligible as compared with that taken for the chemical union of the CO and the hæmoglobin. From the mixing tube the mixture passes along a cylindrical tube at a velocity of the order of 100 cm. per second. The fluid at first does not show the bands of CO-hæmoglobin, but in proportion as the observation-spectroscope is moved further from the mixing chamber so the bands become more intense, until at last the reaction is complete. At last! That is, in about one-tenth of a second with such strengths of solution as were used by Hartridge and Roughton.

Here is a remarkable thing. A few pages back I said that the affinity of carbon monoxide for hæmoglobin was 245 times that of oxygen for hæmoglobin. I said so because hæmoglobin saturates itself equally whether in equilibrium with CO at ·156 mm. pressure or with oxygen at 38 mm. pressure and 38 is 245 times ·156. It would have been natural therefore to expect that the velocity with which carbon monoxide united with hæmoglobin would have been greater than that with which the pigment united with oxygen, but that is not the case. On the other hand, hæmoglobin unites with oxygen ten to twelve times as fast as with carbon monoxide. What is the solution? It is as follows. The pressure of gas at which the hæmoglobin half-saturates itself, and maintains an equilibrium in that condition, depends upon two things, namely, k the velocity with which the hæmoglobin unites with the gas, and k_1 the velocity with which it dissociates from it, and is proportional to the quotient of the two, i.e. to $\frac{k_1}{k}$. When therefore I said that the affinity of hæmoglobin for carbon monoxide was 245 times its affinity for oxygen, I meant that $\frac{k_1 CO}{k_{CO}}$ was 245 times smaller than $\frac{k_1 O_2}{k_{O_2}}$. The statement therefore involved nothing either about the absolute values of k_{CO} and k_{O_2}, or even about their relative values. It means, however, that if k_{CO} is only one-tenth of k_{O_2}, $k_1 CO$ will be but 2450 of $k_{1 O_2}$. In other words, the apparently high affinity of hæmoglobin for carbon monoxide would be due, not to a high velocity constant for the union of CO with hæmoglobin, but to the extreme slowness with which the two separate once they are brought together.

Considerable experimental difficulties attend the measurements both of the association and dissociation velocities. These I touched upon rather lightly a few pages back, because I wished to make clear the theory of what was taking place, without complicating the discussion by the introduction of details of technique. I therefore passed over the method of spectroscopic measurement by saying that the density of the CO-hæmoglobin bands was measured from point to point as the fluid passed along the tube; and that starting from observations taken immediately after the mixed fluid left the mixing chamber, at which point the CO-bands were invisible, the bands became denser as the fluid progressed. Strictly speaking the Hartridge reversion spectroscope does not measure the density of the bands. It measures the shifting of the bands in mixtures of oxy- and carboxy-hæmoglobin according to the relative quantities of the two. But here there is no oxyhæmoglobin. It is possible to attain the object in view, of that of determining the amount of CO-hæmoglobin, by placing a trough of oxyhæmoglobin in the path of the light, so that the observer looks through the optical mixture of a known quantity of oxyhæmoglobin (in the trough) and an unknown quantity of CO-hæmoglobin (in the tube). The position of the bands will tell him the ratio of the one to the other, from which the quantity of CO-hæmoglobin may be deduced. This method of observation, ingenious enough, has the disadvantage of being much less accurate at the ends of the scale than in the middle, i.e. it is unreliable when there is less than 30 per cent. saturation of COHb in the tube and also when there is more than 70 per cent. of CO-hæmoglobin.

To overcome this difficulty the authors adopted a method so bold as to be the admiration of anyone familiar with their type of technique. It was one of those experimental sallies which could only be contemplated by a worker with a complete knowledge of the factors at stake. Instead of putting a layer of oxyhæmoglobin behind the

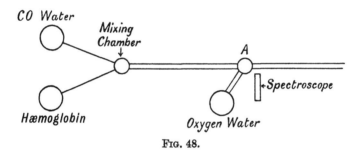

FIG. 48.

observation tube they actually ran oxygen into the tube. Supposing at a certain point A in the tube the reduced hæmoglobin and the CO-hæmoglobin were in the ratio of 30 to 60 per cent., and at that point oxygen water was introduced through a mixing chamber, the oxygen would at once unite with the reduced hæmoglobin, having tenfold the reaction velocity of the carbon monoxide, so that the quantity of carboxyhæmoglobin would be for an instant fixed. In time of course the oxygen would tend to break down the COHb, but for that *time* would be required, and in the interval the spectroscopic observation can be made. The technical difficulties presented by the measurement of the dissociation phase

$$HbCO \longrightarrow Hb + CO$$

are more difficult to overcome, and further work is still to be desired. For instance, the dissociation can only be measured in solutions so dilute that the fluid appears colourless in an ordinary test-tube. The strongest concentration suitable corresponds to about 1 part of blood in 5000 of buffered water. The difficulty is that in order to make the reaction progress in the one direction either or both of the Hb and the CO should be removed as it is formed. The substances tried for the purpose of removing reduced hæmoglobin were oxygen and potassium ferricyanide. The use of oxygen depends for its justification on the assumption that when HbCO in the presence of oxygen forms HbO_2 the reaction consists of two separate stages:

$$HbCO \longrightarrow Hb + CO,$$
$$Hb + O_2 \longrightarrow HbO_2,$$

and not one stage

$$HbCO + O_2 \longrightarrow HbO_2 + CO.$$

Now we shall treat of this reaction in the next chapter, but here we would say that neither view of the nature of the change from carboxy- to oxyhæmoglobin can be regarded as definitely proven. For the view just stated there are several pieces of evidence. Those relevant here are (1) that Hartridge and Roughton did not find increasing the concentration of oxygen appreciably increased the velocity of the decomposition of COHb, and (2) that the maximum rate of dissociation of Hb with CO in the presence of ferricyanide is approximately the same as in the presence of oxygen. The uncertainty of the position prevents us, at present, from adopting any definite coefficient for the dissociation velocity of carboxyhæmoglobin, but it does not obscure the important issue, namely, that the velocity constant is an extremely small one. The breakdown takes place very slowly. Where oxyhæmoglobin would dissociate in a fraction of a second, carboxyhæmoglobin requires minutes, and of these more than one or two. This is so where oxygen is used as a hæmoglobin acceptor. If the use of the oxygen is unjustifiable the reason would be that the oxygen hustled the carbon monoxide out of the hæmoglobin, and the conclusion would be that in the absence of the oxygen the breakdown of the hæmoglobin would be even more leisurely.

Summing up then, if we select conditions of temperature and hydrogen-ion concentration such as are found in the body, we may imagine a certain degree of union of hæmoglobin with oxygen as taking place in one-thousandth of a second; the same degree of union of carbon monoxide with hæmoglobin would take one-hundredth of a second or more. The reverse process in the case of the oxyhæmoglobin would take one-twentieth of a second, and in the case of the CO-hæmoglobin over 3 minutes. The range of Hartridge and

Roughton's work therefore extends to the measurement of velocity coefficients of reactions, one of which is something like two hundred thousand times as rapid as the other.

A moment ago I alluded to conditions of temperature and of hydrogen-ion concentration. Reference to Chapter XI will show that the reaction

$$Hb + O_2 \longrightarrow HbO_2$$

is but slightly affected either by hydrogen-ion concentration or by temperature, but that the reaction

$$HbO_2 \longrightarrow Hb + O_2$$

is extremely sensitive to temperature, and over a certain range of alkalinity to changes in hydrogen-ion concentration. That range is very near the neutral point.

We may ask ourselves: Do these corresponding reactions of hæmoglobin with CO show the same properties? We can speak more confidently about the union of CO and hæmoglobin than about the opposite phase of the reaction. Is it, like that of hæmoglobin with oxygen, independent of temperature and hydrogen-ion concentration? The answer is that both hydrogen-ion concentration and temperature have an influence on the rate of association of carbon monoxide with hæmoglobin, though the influence is not a very great one. Thus the rate of association increases with the alkalinity of the fluid, being about half as great again at $pH = 10$ as at $pH = 6$. Rise of temperature also increases the rate of association of carbon monoxide with hæmoglobin; the velocity constant of the reaction varies from 1·4 to 2 according to the specimen of hæmoglobin studied.

Here therefore are two qualitative differences between the behaviour of hæmoglobin towards carbon monoxide and its behaviour towards oxygen. The other important qualitative difference is that light dissociates carboxyhæmoglobin and not oxyhæmoglobin.

Turning to the dissociation phase of the reaction, it will be recalled that the dissociation of oxyhæmoglobin into reduced hæmoglobin and oxygen has a very high temperature coefficient—in sheep's blood the velocity constant increases about fourfold for a rise of temperature of ten degrees. In the few cases so far observed the temperature coefficient of the dissociation of carboxyhæmoglobin varied between 3 and 6. We have already seen that the velocity of combination of CO with hæmoglobin is scarcely affected by changes in hydrogen-ion concentration. There is a field left for investigation as to why, when the velocity constants of both phases of the reaction are unchanged by cH, the equilibrium constant should have been found, by Barcroft and Murray[6] on hæmoglobin and by Douglas, Haldane and Haldane[1] on whole blood, to have been so greatly influenced.

In many ways the technique associated with research on carboxyhæmoglobin is simpler and runs more rapidly than that which involves oxygen. An estimation with the Hartridge reversion spectroscope takes only a few moments whilst a determination of percentage saturation by gas analysis requires perhaps 45 minutes. Carbon monoxide does not affect a hydrogen electrode as does oxygen, an advantage which has probably disappeared with the introduction of the glass electrode. There is always the chance of adventitious oxidations taking place at the expense of the oxyhæmoglobin, or of the atmosphere to which it is exposed and so forth, and lastly, in the case of dilute solutions of oxyhæmoglobin, it can scarcely be said that methods exist of estimating the percentage saturation over the whole range of a dissociation curve from 0 to − 100 per cent.

There has always been the hope therefore that the more important facts regarding hæmoglobin were to be obtained more easily by a study of the carboxy- than of the oxy- body, and that having been found out on CO-hæmoglobin, the results could be transferred bodily to oxyhæmoglobin.

It was this hope which inspired the following technique. A given quantity of a dilute solution of carboxyhæmoglobin is put into each of a series of saturators of very different sizes.

Suppose 5 c.c. of a solution of hæmoglobin made by diluting blood fifty times are used, and the blood has a CO capacity of 1 c.c. = ·190 c.c. of CO, then 5 c.c. of the dilute solution will have a CO capacity of $\frac{·190}{50} \times 5 = ·019$ c.c. This is then put into a saturator which contains hydrogen which is free from any trace either of carbon monoxide or of oxygen. Now if this tonometer is shaken sufficiently and if all goes well, some of the CO will be shaken out and an equilibrium will be established. Suppose at the end an estimation shows that the hæmoglobin is 40 per cent. reduced Hb and 60 per cent. COHb, clearly $\frac{60}{100} \times ·019$ c.c. of CO will have been ceded to the atmosphere.

If this atmosphere occupies a volume of 5 litres the pressure of CO will be $\frac{·019 \times 60}{100} \times \frac{760}{5000}$ mm. = ·0017 mm. Thus a single measurement will give both the percentage saturation and the CO-pressure. The use of 5 tonometers will give five points on a curve, and other points may be obtained by varying the amount of hæmoglobin solution which is used. In our experiments the tonometers are made so that 5, 10 or 15 c.c. of fluid can easily be measured into them.

Even this simple technique bristles with difficulties—chiefly those which only appear when an effort is made to obtain real accuracy. This was found to be so by Hecht, and confirmed by Forbes and Morgan[7], who for a year devoted the most untiring energy (to use a rhetorical phrase, for by the time the vacation came they each required a rest-

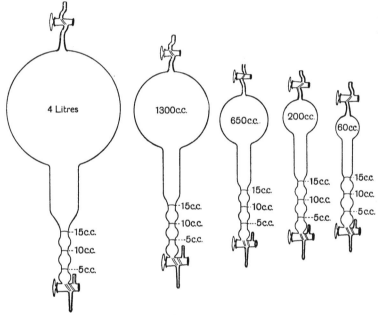

FIG. 49.

cure) to the method. The difficulty of being certain of an equilibrium could be overcome with ease, for it was possible either to strike it from above simply by shaking out the CO, or to strike it from below by driving out all the CO and allowing the hæmoglobin to unite again with the gas. The expulsion of the CO from the hæmoglobin is effected by a strong light.

It soon appeared that the reversion spectroscope as ordinarily used was not sufficiently accurate for the purpose, though more accurate in most peoples' hands than any previous method for the estimation of carboxyhæmoglobin. The possibility of using spectrophotographic methods was discussed, but finally Hecht decided to make use of a photographic method which had been worked out by Hartridge and Roughton (8) for another purpose. For this purpose the mixture of CO and reduced hæmoglobin is taken into a trough, protected from air and a measured quantity of aerated water added to convert the

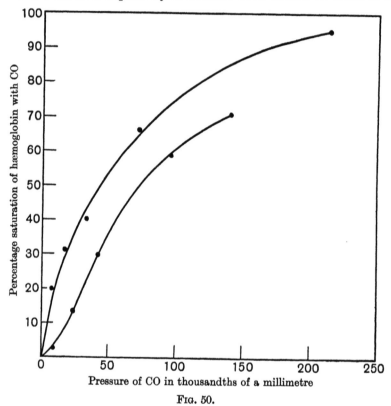

Fig. 50.

reduced hæmoglobin into oxyhæmoglobin. The spectrum is then photographed under standard conditions and the proportion of CO estimated from the photographic plate by analysis with the densitometer.

This technique, so far as the making of all the estimations is concerned, is in many ways a decided advance on any of its predecessors. The improvement was aptly expressed by someone who, looking at one of Hecht and Morgan's curves, said, "This is the first dissociation curve I have seen where the points really lie on the curve."

Having overcome the difficulties of estimation there remain others of a much more subtle character. Of these one was pointed out by Douglas, Haldane and Haldane[1] in the following words: "Violent shaking had to be avoided on account of its effect in producing mechanical coagulation, but satisfactory saturation could easily be

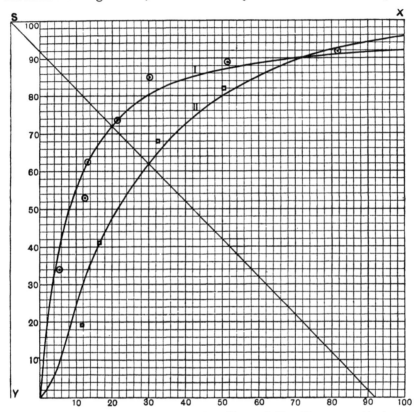

Fig. 51. Ordinates = percentage saturation of hæmoglobin with oxygen. Abscissæ = tension of oxygen in mm. of mercury. Curve I = rectangular hyperbola. $XY = 800$. Curve II = Bohr's dissociation curve of hæmoglobin.
⊙ Points determined from dialysed solution.
□ Points determined from undialysed solution.

obtained by rotating the blood in a saturator." Now the pressures of carbon monoxide with which Douglas, Haldane and Haldane worked were measured in tenths of a millimetre, those with which Hecht and Morgan worked were measured in hundredths or thousandths of a millimetre, therefore the latter workers could not avoid violent shaking, but by buffering the solution well on the alkaline side of neutral ($pH = 11$) they avoided mechanical coagulation, as indeed the Oxford workers had done by the addition of ammonia.

Hitherto this technique has brought us nearer finality chiefly by revealing a fresh source of uncertainty. It would appear that when kept under the most rigorous conditions, i.e. at $- 1°$ C., even a solution of hæmoglobin which has been crystallised alters in the following way: the dissociation curve approximates more nearly to a hyperbola as time goes on. Fig. 50 shows the result of time, even in the cold, on such a solution. There are on it two curves, taken from the same solution of hæmoglobin, the first 58 hours, the second 5 days after dialysis. It is evident that the double inflection is almost gone from the older hæmoglobin.

The curves drawn represent dissociation curves derived from Hill's equation with values of 1·4 and 1·2 respectively for the "n's" of the less and more "matured" solutions. How like is Fig. 50 to one of our oldest friends—Fig. 51!

REFERENCES

(1) DOUGLAS, HALDANE, J. B. S. AND HALDANE, J. S. *Journ. Physiol.* XLIV. 275. 1912.

(2) BOHR, HASSELBALCH AND KROGH. *Skand. Arch. f. Physiol.* XVI. 390. 1907.

(3) PARSONS, T. R. *Journ. Physiol.* LI. 440. 1917.

(4) HASTINGS, SENDROY, MURRAY AND HEIDELBERGER. *Journ. Biol. Chem.* LXI. 317. 1924.

(5) HARTRIDGE AND ROUGHTON. (As yet unpublished.)

(6) BARCROFT AND MURRAY. Appendix to "Observations upon the Effect of High Altitudes,...chiefly at Cerro de Pasco." *Phil. Trans. Roy. Soc.* B. CCXI. 351. 1923.

(7) HECHT, MORGAN AND FORBES. (As yet unpublished.)

(8) HARTRIDGE AND ROUGHTON. (As yet unpublished.)

CHAPTER XV

THE INTERACTION OF CARBON MONOXIDE AND OXYGEN WITH HÆMOGLOBIN

THE precise nature of this interaction between oxygen, carbon monoxide and hæmoglobin is at present a matter on which no certain statement can be made. The reaction has usually been treated as though it were represented by the following equation:

$$HbCO + O_2 \rightleftarrows HbO_2 + CO.$$

There is, however (as pointed out by Hartridge and Roughton[1]), another possibility, namely, that the so-called reaction is really a series of two reactions, namely,

(a) $HbCO \rightleftarrows Hb + CO,$
(b) $Hb + O_2 \rightleftarrows HbO_2.$

The evidence, so far as it goes, will now be given briefly.

The positive evidence in favour of the reaction of hæmoglobin with oxygen and carbon monoxide, being two separate reactions which take place successively but independently rather than being a double decomposition, may be considered under two headings, firstly, as regards the conversion of carboxyhæmoglobin into oxyhæmoglobin, and secondly, the conversion of oxy- into carboxyhæmoglobin.

I. On this theory the first of these would be represented as follows:

(a) $HbCO \longrightarrow CO + Hb,$
(b) $Hb + O_2 \longrightarrow HbO_2.$

Indeed, even that is only a partial picture of this conception of the reaction, for the phase (a) is so much slower than the phase (b) that the reduced hæmoglobin and the oxygen may always be regarded as being in equilibrium, standing at attention, so to speak, and waiting for a little more Hb to be liberated; so that the velocity of the reaction is entirely controlled by the velocity of phase (a).

The evidence for the reaction:

(a) $HbCO \longrightarrow CO + Hb,$
(b) $Hb + O_2 \rightleftarrows HbO_2,$

rather than

$$HbCO + O_2 \longrightarrow HbO_2 + CO,$$

has been given in the last chapter, and is briefly that oxygen or ferricyanide can be used as acceptors of the hæmoglobin without retarding the rate at which the HbCO is broken down.

II. So much for the conversion of carboxyhæmoglobin into oxy-hæmoglobin; now as regards the opposite phase, the conversion of the oxy- into the carboxy-compound. Here again, if there are two stages in the reaction:

$$(a) \quad HbO_2 \quad \rightleftharpoons O_2 + Hb,$$
$$(b) \quad Hb + CO \longrightarrow HbCO,$$

the first is much more rapid than the second, though the disparity is not so great as in the previous case, so that here also the oxygen and the reduced hæmoglobin are practically in equilibrium, and the rate at which the whole process proceeds is governed principally by the rate at which reduced hæmoglobin unites with carbon monoxide; nevertheless it is to some extent influenced by the rate at which the hæmoglobin is liberated. Now if the reaction were

$$HbO_2 + CO \longrightarrow HbCO + O_2$$

the velocity *in that direction* would be influenced only by the reacting masses of the HbO_2 and CO and not at all by the active masses of the O_2 or of the HbCO. Of course as these last accumulate they would set up a reaction in the opposite direction, but that is another matter.

Now, in practice, the velocity of the reaction in the direction from HbO_2 to HbCO does depend on the reacting mass of oxygen, and this is intelligible on the two-stage theory, for the increase in the reacting mass of oxygen, by pushing the reaction (a) in the direction

$$HbO_2 \longleftarrow O_2 + Hb,$$

will decrease the concentration of Hb at any given time and therefore decrease the active mass of Hb available for the reaction (b).

So much for the evidence in favour of the two-stage reaction: now as to the difficulties regarding it.

As a preliminary it may be useful to tabulate the effects of increased hydrogen-ion concentration and temperature on the principal reactions which have been considered. (See table on p. 163.)

Now if the conversion from oxy- to carboxyhæmoglobin is in two stages, following equations (2) and (3) in the table below, the effects of temperature and pH should be the products of the individual coefficients, i.e. a rise of 10° C. should accelerate the reaction between $4 \times 1\cdot4$ and 4×2-fold, but in point of fact the velocity is only increased 2–3-fold. Again an increase of hydrogen-ion concentration from pH 10 to pH 6 should increase the velocity not less than $6 \times 1\cdot5$ times, but in reality the effect of increased hydrogen-ion concentration is almost negligible (2), (3).

Reaction	Effect of pH between pH 6 and pH 10	Temperature coefficient over 10° C.
(1) Hb + O$_2$ —→ HbO$_2$ ...	1·5	1–1·5
(2) HbO$_2$ —→ Hb + O$_2$ ...	6–10	4
(3) Hb + CO —→ HbCO ...	1·5	1·4–2
(4) HbCO —→ Hb + CO ...	1	3–6
(5) HbCO + O$_2$ —→ HbO$_2$ + CO	1	3–6
(6) HbO$_2$ + CO —→ HbCO + O$_2$	1	2–3

There is another difficulty also, namely, that the reaction

$$HbO_2 + CO \longrightarrow HbCO + O_2$$

proceeds on the average at more than twice the velocity calculated from the individual velocity coefficients of the two stages.

The study of that reaction (observed first by Haldane (2) and confirmed by Hartridge (3)) formed the starting-point of Hartridge and Roughton's work. Their method briefly was to dissociate carboxyhæmoglobin by light in the presence of oxygen and then to observe the rate at which the COHb was re-formed.

The effect of light upon carboxyhæmoglobin is no haphazard affair. In a system which consists of O$_2$, CO, oxy- and carboxyhæmoglobins an equilibrium is always being maintained between these four substances, which behaves quantitatively as though it were expressed by the equation

$$HbCO + O_2 \rightleftarrows HbO_2 + CO.$$

When light of definite brightness shines on a solution containing the above substances, a fresh equilibrium is established, so that more HbO$_2$ and less HbCO is in the solution. When the bright light is turned off the CO which has been displaced reunites with the hæmoglobin, the rate of this reunion can be measured, and therefore the velocity constant of the reaction

$$HbO_2 + CO \longrightarrow HbCO + O_2$$

can be calculated.

However doubtful may be the exact nature of the process which accounts for the partition of hæmoglobin between oxygen and carbon monoxide, certain properties of the reaction are amongst the best established facts with which we have to deal.

Of these we may commence with the shape of the curve which forms the graphic representation of the reaction. This curve is a rectangular hyperbola, as was proved by Haldane and Lorrain Smith (4). But the interesting point with regard to it is that while the evidence in favour of the curve being a rectangular hyperbola seemed to be very good, the precise position of the curve was a matter of some doubt.

In Fig. 52 is shown Haldane and Lorrain Smith's curve (1897). The ordinate of this curve requires no special discussion. If the whole quantity of hæmoglobin is called 100, the figure at any point indicates the percentage of that hæmoglobin which is saturated with carbon monoxide, it being always assumed that the remainder is saturated with oxygen and therefore that no appreciable quantity of reduced hæmoglobin is present. The abscissa of the curve requires careful consideration. The figures along it are as given in Haldane and Lorrain Smith's paper and consist of "percentages of carbon monoxide in air"—this fact may be grasped without a full understanding of its significance, for it is implicit in the figures that 21 per cent. of oxygen is present the whole time. The figures therefore are not absolute quantities of CO but, like those standing against the ordinate, they are really ratios and mean if fully written out:

$$\frac{CO}{O_2} = \frac{\cdot 05}{21}, \frac{\cdot 1}{21}, \text{etc.}$$

In theory there is an error involved in spacing out equally the figures $\cdot 1$, $\cdot 2$, $\cdot 3$, etc. per cent. of CO in air because if you dilute the air with CO you reduce the quantity of oxygen present, and therefore if the curve commences at

$$\frac{CO}{O_2} = \frac{0}{21},$$

it would end as shown on the paper with

$$\frac{CO}{O_2} = \frac{\cdot 5}{21 \times \frac{99 \cdot 5}{100}},$$

the air being diluted to the extent of $\cdot 5$ parts in 100. In practice the error is so small as not to matter. But it is possible to draw the

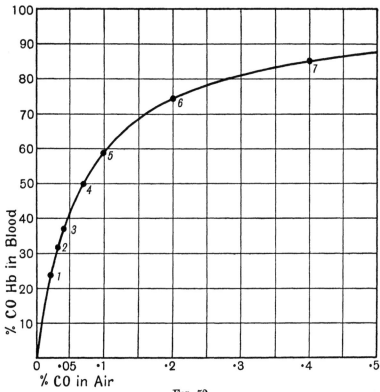

FIG. 52.

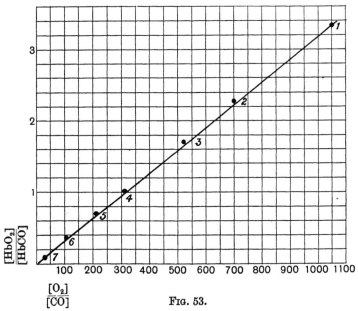

FIG. 53.

curve in a way which really expresses what the curve means. If we plot along the ordinate the relative concentrations of oxy- to carboxyhæmoglobin, starting from zero and extending to infinity, and plot along the abscissa the relative concentrations of oxygen to carbon monoxide in the air to which the hæmoglobin is exposed also starting from zero, the curve given above would be transformed as follows. Taking the points as numbered in Fig. 52, 1, 2, etc., we read:

Serial number of point...	1	2	3	4	5	6	7
Percentage HbCO	23	31	37	50	59	74	85
Percentage CO in air ...	·02	·03	·04	·068	·10	·20	·40

Now to make the transformation we may select the first point, 23 per cent. of HbCO means 77 per cent. of HbO_2, therefore the ratio $\dfrac{HbO_2}{HbCO}$ is $\dfrac{77}{23} = 3\cdot33$. This is read along the ordinate (Fig. 53). The percentage of CO in air is ·02, the ratio therefore of O_2 to CO is $\dfrac{21}{\cdot02} = 1050$. This is plotted along the abscissa. The result is the point labelled 1 in Fig. 53, and so with the other points. We therefore obtain the following data:

Serial number of point...			1	2	3	4	5	6	7
A. Ratio $\dfrac{O_2}{CO}$ ...	...		1050	700	525	310	210	105	52·5
B. Ratio $\dfrac{HbO_2}{HbCO}$		...	3·33	2·23	1·7	1	0·69	0·35	·017
$\dfrac{A}{B}$	...	...	...	306	314	310	310	304	300	310

This method of plotting has many advantages over that given in Fig. 52. It enables the reader much more easily to understand the real properties of the reaction.

The first point to which attention may be drawn is that at which the hæmoglobin is half-oxy- and half-carboxyhæmoglobin, and at which the ratio $\dfrac{[HbO_2]}{[HbCO]} = 1$ (see point 4). At that point the relative concentrations of oxygen and CO in the air are $\dfrac{[O_2]}{[CO]} = 310 : 1$. The first thing to note then is that the carbon monoxide is 310 times as strong as the oxygen, inasmuch as that in 1/310 of the concentration it will grasp an equal quantity of hæmoglobin.

The next point is that whilst the quotient of the abscissa divided by the ordinate (310 ÷ 1) naturally is 310, the quotient of the distance of any other point on the curve from the abscissa and ordinate is also 310; we may express it thus for the whole curve

$$\frac{[O_2]}{[CO]} \times \frac{[HbCO]}{[HbO_2]} = 310.$$

This is conditioned by the fact that the curve is a hyperbola, and in so far as it is not true of the actual figures given for the points tabulated above, the error is due to the fact that they are read from a diagram, i.e. to the fallibility of human drawing.

Thirdly, if

$$\frac{[O_2]}{[CO]} \times \frac{[HbCO]}{[HbO_2]} = 310,$$

it follows that

$$\frac{[HbCO]}{[HbO_2]} = 310 \frac{[CO]}{[O_2]}.$$

Not merely one point on the curve—that at which the oxy- and carboxyhæmoglobin are present in equal quantities—but every point on the curve is defined by the number 310, because at every point the ratio of carboxy- to oxyhæmoglobin is 310 times the ratio of carbon monoxide to oxygen.

The figure 310 is in fact the equilibrium constant of the reaction and is usually denoted by the letter K.

To retrace our steps. I said a while ago that Haldane and his associates found a number of curves, with somewhat different values of K, each of which appeared to represent the equilibrium between oxygen, carbon monoxide and hæmoglobin. It was a matter of some interest to discover why such differences should exist. At first the presumption was in favour of some sort of experimental error, such for instance as insufficient time given for the equilibration of the blood. The acceptance in 1909 of the general view that changes in hydrogen-ion concentration, temperature and saline content of hæmoglobin solutions, altered the dissociation curve of oxyhæmoglobin, made it more reasonable to believe that the various curves which had been obtained for the reaction

$$HbCO + O_2 \rightleftharpoons CO + HbO_2$$

were *not* merely due to experimental error, but to more substantial causes. To quote Douglas, Haldane and Haldane [2]:

The influence of CO_2 and that of salts on the curve were also quite unsuspected. The researches of Zuntz and Loewy, Bohr and Barcroft and their associates, have, however, altered completely the current conceptions of the dissociation of oxy-hæmoglobin and this fact alone rendered a further investigation of Haldane and Lorrain Smith's conclusions very desirable....And Dr Krogh[5] had also kindly informed us by letter that he had obtained results different from those of Haldane and Lorrain Smith when he used the blood of a different animal.

The necessity of undertaking this work was as evident in Cambridge as in Oxford and therefore it happened that quite independently the equilibrium between CO, O_2 and hæmoglobin was investigated both by the authors just quoted and by Hartridge[3]. Both published their results in 1912.

These researches agreed that alterations of hydrogen-ion concentration had no influence upon the relative affinities of O_2 and CO for hæmoglobin. The following table, given by Hartridge, aptly illustrates the point:

CO-hæmoglobin in tubes containing various concentrations of CO in air

	A	B	C	D	E
No lactic acid	23·5	40·5	54	62	34·5
·075 % lactic acid	23·5	40	55	63	34
·025 % lactic acid	23·2	41·5	59	63	35

In each column the gas mixture is the same for the three samples.

The Oxford observers, who determined the CO-O_2-Hb dissociation curve with hæmoglobin to which CO_2 and Na_2CO_3 had been added, similarly found that neither the CO_2 nor the Na_2CO_3 had any appreciable influence on the result.

Salts also appear to have no effect on the equilibrium. With temperature it is otherwise. Temperature has a definite effect on the reaction, though this effect is trifling as compared with the effect of temperature on the affinity of hæmoglobin for either gas separately. Thus, according to the determinations of Haldane and his collaborators, the equilibrium constant of human hæmoglobin at 37° C. is 250, at 15° C. it is 400—an alteration of 10–20 per cent. for a change of temperature of 10°; it will be remembered that the equilibrium constant of the reaction

$$Hb + O_2 \rightleftarrows HbO$$

has a temperature coefficient of about 400 per cent. over the same range of temperature.

Whilst the factors which influence the reaction of hæmoglobin with oxygen have little influence on the equilibrium of hæmoglobin with the oxygen and carbon monoxide simultaneously, there is another factor, namely, light, to which the reaction is very sensitive. Light tends to expel the CO from hæmoglobin to the advantage of the oxygen. If, therefore, the equilibrium between oxygen and hæmoglobin and CO is struck in the light, there will be a less percentage of CO-hæmoglobin and a greater percentage of oxyhæmoglobin, than if the equilibrium is struck in the dark. So far as I know no systematic work has been published on this subject, in the sense that the quantitative relation of the value of K to the measured intensity of light has never been determined even for any specified wave length; but the general effect has been observed by many who have worked upon the subject—Haldane in the first instance and later Hartridge and others. The subject will be more fully discussed in a later chapter.

In the above discussion of the reaction of hæmoglobin with oxygen and carbon monoxide simultaneously it has been assumed tacitly that sufficient of the two gases taken together has been available for the saturation of the hæmoglobin with either the one or the other, that is to say that no appreciable amount of reduced hæmoglobin is present. The consideration of the system, Hb, HbO_2, HbCO, O_2 and CO, all present simultaneously, forms a very interesting problem and one on which little work has been done.

The following avenue of approach might seem to be a rather natural view of the subject, and one which has been used by Douglas, Haldane and Haldane[2] and A. V. Hill[6].

Consider first the quantity of reduced hæmoglobin in the system; a curve may be drawn indicating the quantity of hæmoglobin which is not combined with gas, from that which is. The gas pressure may be expressed in equivalents of oxygen pressure; reverting to the example given on page 166, one part of CO would count as 310 equivalents of oxygen. So that a mixture of ·01 mm. of CO and 5 mm. of O_2 would count as

$$CO = ·01 \times 310 = 3·1$$
$$O_2 = 5 \qquad = 5$$
$$\overline{8·1}\text{ virtual mm. } O_2.$$

The dissociation curve then between gas-free and gas-combined hæmoglobin would be the ordinary one of oxyhæmoglobin, but in which mm. O_2-pressure was replaced by virtual mm. O_2-pressure.

The partition of the gas-combined hæmoglobin would then take place just as if the reduced hæmoglobin were not present. To carry the examples given above a little further.

Assuming, for the sake of argument, the dissociation curve of Barcroft and Roberts for dialysed hæmoglobin, 8·1 virtual mm. of oxygen would correspond to 51 per cent. of gas-combined hæmoglobin and 49 per cent. of reduced hæmoglobin. Of the 51 per cent. of gas-combined hæmoglobin how much is oxy- and how much is carboxyhæmoglobin?

$$\frac{[O_2]}{[CO]} = \frac{5}{\cdot 01} = 500;$$

from Fig. 53 it appears that

$$\frac{[HbO_2]}{[HbCO]} \text{ will therefore be } \frac{1\cdot 6}{1}.$$

Therefore out of 2·6 parts of hæmoglobin 1·6 will be HbO_2 and 1·0 will be HbCO, out of 51 parts 31·4 will be HbO_2 and 19·6 will be HbCO, so that the whole hæmoglobin would be divided as follows (Fig. 54):

Reduced hæmoglobin ...	49	parts
Oxyhæmoglobin ...	31·4	,,
CO-hæmoglobin ...	19·6	,,
Total hæmoglobin	100	,,

Or to take another example, suppose hæmoglobin is exposed to a mixture of 20 mm. O_2 and ·032 mm. CO. The CO corresponds to ·032 × 310 = 10 virtual mm. of oxygen, making the equivalent of 30 oxygen mm. That on the curve would correspond to 20 per cent. of reduced hæmoglobin and 80 per cent. of a mixture of oxy- and carboxyhæmoglobin. The proportion of these last to one another is found in Fig. 53 which really amounts to this:

$$\frac{[HbO_2]}{[HbCO]} = \frac{\text{Pressure of } O_2}{\text{Pressure of CO expressed in virtual mm. of } O_2}.$$

Therefore the

$$\frac{[HbO_2]}{[HbCO]} = \frac{20}{10},$$

so that of the whole hæmoglobin:

Reduced hæmoglobin	20	per cent.
$HbO_2 = \frac{20}{30} \times 80$	53	,,
$HbCO = \frac{10}{30} \times 80$	27	,,
Total hæmoglobin	100	,,

It will be observed that in both the cases I have given there is less, both of oxy- and of carboxyhæmoglobin, than if reduced hæmoglobin had been exposed to the existing pressure either of oxygen or CO in the absence of the other. Thus 20 mm. pressure of oxygen alone would have produced 68 and not 53 per cent. of oxyhæmoglobin while CO, to the extent of 10 virtual mm. of oxygen, would have produced 55 and not 27 per cent. of HbCO. Similarly at the point lower down the curve 5 mm. of oxygen alone would have produced

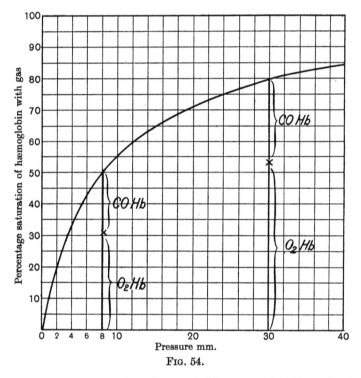

Fig. 54.

38 and not 31 per cent. of oxyhæmoglobin, and CO to the extent of 3·1 virtual mm. of O_2 would have produced about 27 per cent. of HbCO and not 9·8 per cent. That seems all straightforward and as it should be.

I must now break it to the reader that I was guilty of some degree of subtlety in selecting the hyperbolic dissociation curve as the basis of my calculations, for had I chosen the dissociation curve of blood we should have been faced at the outset with certain anomalies which I will now proceed to describe: they are of considerable interest.

Consider the last of the two examples given, 20 mm. O_2 and CO equivalent to 10 mm. of oxygen. Applying these figures to the ordinary dissociation curve of blood (at 40 mm. CO_2-pressure and

37° C.), the reduced hæmoglobin amounts to 48 per cent., the oxy- + carboxy- to 52 per cent., and as before two-thirds of this will be oxyhæmoglobin and one-third carboxyhæmoglobin, so that the final composition of the mixture would be (Fig. 55):

Reduced hæmoglobin	48	per cent.
Oxyhæmoglobin	35	,,
Carboxyhæmoglobin	17	,,
Total hæmoglobin	100	,,

Here is the apparent anomaly. Twenty mm. of oxygen pressure in the absence of CO would only produce 27 per cent. of oxyhæmoglobin,

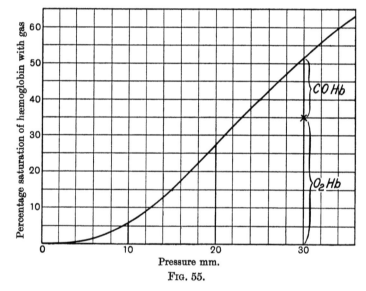

FIG. 55.

not 35 per cent. CO equivalent to 10 mm. of oxygen would only produce 6 per cent. of HbCO, not 17 per cent. Therefore the mixture of oxyhæmoglobin and carboxyhæmoglobin is richer in either of the two, if the CO and O_2 are presented simultaneously, than would be the case if O_2 or CO were in equilibrium with hæmoglobin in the absence of the other.

A few examples will show the reader, if it is not already apparent to him, that this paradox is essentially due to the concavity (viewed from the ordinate) of the lower part of the dissociation curve. Such a paradox might well shake one's faith in the whole method of treatment adopted, namely, that of regarding the reactions of hæmoglobin with oxygen and with CO as independent of one another, were it not for the fact that (according to Douglas, Haldane and Haldane) the paradox actually is the expression of the experimental facts.

Fig. 56, which is a portion of Fig. 7, page 292, of their paper, shows the percentage saturation of the blood with CO. Each line represents a certain pressure of CO which for that line remains constant. That pressure would, if there were no oxygen present, saturate the blood to the degree indicated at the intersection of the line in question

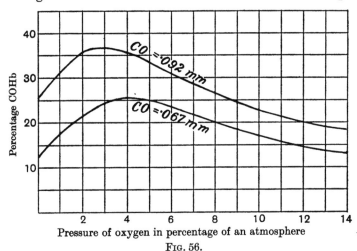

Pressure of oxygen in percentage of an atmosphere

Fig. 56.

with the ordinate. The abscissa represents the amount of oxygen present. On the curves a little oxygen increases the quantities of carboxyhæmoglobin present. If, and when, we are able to get a dissociation curve for the equilibrium

$$CO + Hb \rightleftharpoons HbCO$$

(and for the corresponding reaction for oxygen), which is a hyperbola, it will be interesting to see whether this curious property will disappear as in theory it should.

REFERENCES

(1) HARTRIDGE AND ROUGHTON. Communication to Physiol. Soc. May 1925.

(2) DOUGLAS, HALDANE, J. B. S. AND HALDANE, J. S. *Journ. Physiol.* XLIV. 275. 1913.

(3) HARTRIDGE. *Journ. Physiol.* XLIV. 23. 1913.

(4) HALDANE AND LORRAIN SMITH. *Journ. Physiol.* XXII. 231. 1897.

(5) KROGH. Published later in *Skand. Arch. f. Physiol.* XXIII. 217. 1910.

(6) HILL, A. V. *Journ. Biol. Chem.* LI. 359. 1922.

CHAPTER XVI

THE EFFECT OF TEMPERATURE ON HÆMOGLOBIN

A FRIEND of mine once said to me, concerning a certain book, that he liked to give it to his pupils to read because it showed that quite important discoveries could be made as the result of mental processes of a not very high order. I never think of that remark without feeling a secret hope that he did not know how I came to investigate the effect of temperature on hæmoglobin. Of course I know how I should have come to take the matter up. I should have known that oxyhæmoglobin was an exothermic compound, I should from that have gone on to reason that rise of temperature would have weakened the link between hæmoglobin and oxygen, I might then from the published data on the heat of formation of oxyhæmoglobin have endeavoured to apply Van t' Hoff's equation and discovered what might be the difference in the equilibrium constants of the reactions between hæmoglobin and oxygen at different temperatures; all this might have involved "mental processes of a not very high order," but it would at least have been a respectable way of approaching the subject.

The actual avenue was far otherwise. Dr Camis and I were working out an oxygen dissociation curve for which purpose we were equilibrating some hæmoglobin in the crude way in which we did things in those days—just corking up some hæmoglobin in a glass tube with the necessary atmosphere and shaking the tube in a water bath heated with an ordinary gas flame. Well, on this occasion someone came into the laboratory and interrupted me, so that I left the tube in the bath. I came back to find that the temperature had risen about three or four degrees (Centigrade). The point, when plotted, also to my chagrin, did not fall on the same curve as its fellows. I did it over again, this time keeping the bath at constant temperature, and at the second attempt the point fell into line. So I discarded the first point for the time being; but I did put the record of it into a drawer, and on a subsequent occasion I made the definite comparison of two curves drawn on the same blood but at different temperatures. Comparison of these curves is to be found in the paper by W. O. R. King and myself in Vol. xxxix of the *Journal of Physiology* (1).

Yet these early experiments, with all their crudities, have their merits, which curiously enough turn on the very absence of mental processes involved in their conduct, whether these processes be of a high or low order. I often wonder at the frequency with which I turn back to some of the pages in Vols. xxxix and xlii of the *Journal of Physiology*, as compared with those of later papers. And the reason is that the curves given in those papers were made without any preconceived idea about what shape they ought to be if this or that theory were true, or if the views of *A* were to be preferred to those of *B*. And so it was a matter of curiosity to me to see what I made of the dissociation curves of oxyhæmoglobin at different temperatures when I did not know what sort of shape a dissociation curve ought to be, and whether temperature had any effect at all. Of course I should have known, for Paul Bert (2), with that wonderful vision which so far outran the experimental methods of his day, had made some observations on the subject. At room temperature he found that *blood* at 15 mm. oxygen pressure was 90 per cent. saturated with oxygen, whereas at body temperature it was but 50 per cent. saturated. That observation of course contains the kernel of the thing, although it was not made at any specified carbonic acid pressure or anything of that kind. Hüfner (3) also, in 1889, made some observations which tended in the same direction.

But to return. Brown and Hill (4)[1], who studied the effect of temperature on the dissociation curve of blood, have produced a very beautiful series of dissociation curves which *as curves for blood* will become classical: they do not serve our present purpose, however, which is concerned not with blood but with hæmoglobin. We must go back and consider the earlier data of Barcroft and Hill (5). Their curves do not take us any further because it was assumed that the curves were hyperbolic and on that assumption it was considered only necessary to determine one point on each curve, and from that point to draw the curve. Therefore we get back to the original curves of Barcroft and King, which I had always regarded as too crude to

---

[1] The essential difficulty in the application of curves such as Brown and Hill's (in which the temperature varies greatly while the CO_2-pressure is constant) to hæmoglobin is as follows: as the temperature rises the amount of combined CO_2 alters but little whilst the amount of free CO_2 becomes much reduced. Hence the higher the temperature the more alkaline the blood.

be helpful in any theoretical treatment of the subject. Only recently for the first time had I the curiosity to turn back to these curves and see what they really looked like in the light of later-day tests.

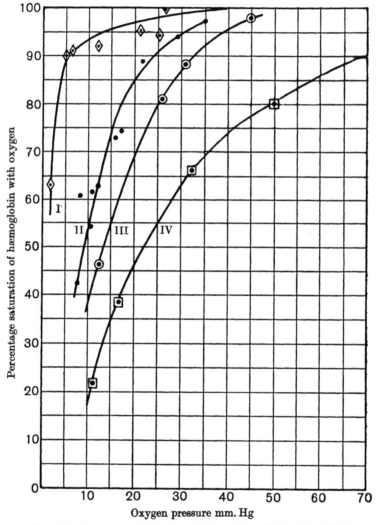

FIG. 57. Curve I at 14° C., II at 26° C., III at 32° C., IV at 38° C.

Fig. 57 shows the points obtained by King and myself. The lines are the same as those in our original figure except that (1) the one corresponding to 38° C. has been drawn more rigidly through the points (this line, as stated in Barcroft and King's paper, was Bohr's line (6) which nearly fitted the points), and (2) the considerable extra-polated portions have been cut off, except at the top of the 38° line, where we have Bohr's work to guide us.

Now as regards the relation of these curves to one another: imagine five horizontal lines drawn corresponding to saturations 90, 80, 64, 50 and 40 per cent. The pressures at which the curves intersect these horizontals are as follows:

Curve	Pressures in mm. corresponding to saturations stated			
	14° C.	26° C.	32° C.	38° C.
Percentage saturation 90	5	24·5	33	72
,, 80	3·5	17	26	49
,, 64	2	12·5	17	31
,, 50	—	8	12	21
,, 40	—	7	11	18

If now each of these pressures be expressed as a percentage of the pressure at 38° C. for the same saturation the table appears as follows:

Curve	Pressures expressed as percentages of the pressure for the same saturation at 38° C.			
	14° C.	26° C.	32° C.	38° C.
Percentage saturation 90	7	34	46	100
,, 80	7	35	53	100
,, 64	6·5	38	55	100
,, 50	—	38	57	100
,, 40	—	39	61	100

The identity of the above percentage pressures for the various lines is, I think, quite remarkable and certainly the variations are not greater than the experimental errors involved. The greatest deviation is the lower portion of the 32° line. This deviation depends upon one point, an error of 1 mm. in the pressure of that point would bring it into good agreement with the rest.

The curves all seem to be of the same degree of inflection (in Hill's notation $n = 1·8$ approximately): we may therefore proceed to consider the implication of that fact. I am indebted to Adair for the following statement of the fact that identity of inflection is irreconcilable with any view of the essence of the reaction between oxygen and hæmoglobin other than that of its being a chemical combination:

Thermodynamical reasoning shows that if the pressure of oxygen required to keep an hæmoglobin solution at a constant degree of saturation is equal to p_1 when the temperature is T_1, and the pressure required to maintain the same degree of saturation is p_2 when the temperature is T_2, the heat of reaction (Q) per gram mol. of oxygen is given by the formula below:

$$Q = 2{\cdot}303 \times R \times \frac{T_1 T_2}{T_1 - T_2} \times \log \frac{p_2}{p_1}.$$

This equation is independent of the mechanism of the reaction—it applies to the heats of adsorption of gases on charcoal as well as to chemical reactions.

There is, however, an important difference between the heats of adsorption and the heat of reaction of hæmoglobin.

In adsorption Q is large at low saturations with gas and it diminishes as the pressure is increased. In the case of hæmoglobin, increase of temperature alters the scale of the curve but not its shape. That is to say, the ratio $\frac{p_1}{p_2}$ at a low saturation is the same as the ratio $\frac{p_1}{p_2}$ measured for a higher saturation, and according to the thermodynamic formula, the heat of reaction Q must be the same at all degrees of oxygenation. This conclusion applies to blood and to certain hæmoglobin solutions, but it does not necessarily apply to solutions in which a large change in pH takes place on oxygenation.

To pass to another point. Granting that the only difference between the curves in Fig. 57 is the horizontal scale on which they are drawn we may proceed to consider some other of their properties. The pressures at which the hæmoglobin is 50 per cent. saturated are for the temperatures given as follows:

| Temperature (° C.) ... ... | 14 | 26 | 32 | 38 |
| Pressure for half-saturation (mm.) | 2 | 8 | 11 | 22 |

These pressures are related to the equilibrium constants of the reaction. In Henderson's[7] view they would be proportional to the equilibrium constants K, for the various temperatures, in Hill's they would be proportional to the reciprocals of $\sqrt[n]{K}$ in his equation.

In either case we should be able to find the heat evolved when one molecule of oxygen unites with hæmoglobin (according to Henderson's view with one molecule, according to Hill's view with $\frac{1}{n}$ molecule of hæmoglobin).

If these pressures be considered proportional to the equilibrium constants of the reactions of oxygen with hæmoglobin (i.e. the velocity of association divided by the velocity of dissociation—the equilibrium constant in Hill's equation is the reciprocal of this) it is possible to work out from them the temperature coefficient of the reactions. This is done most simply by plotting the logarithms of the 50/50 pressures against the reciprocal of the absolute temperatures. The result is given in Fig. 58.

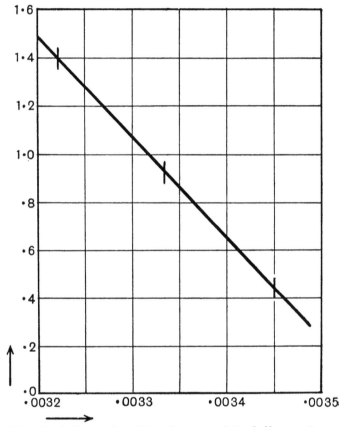

FIG. 58.   Ordinate = logarithm of pressure giving half-saturation.
Abscissa = reciprocal of absolute temperature.

Over a range of ten degrees, between 17° C. and 27° C., the temperature coefficient is 3·2 and between 27° C. and 37° C. the temperature coefficient is 2·8. At this distance of time I cannot remember, if indeed I knew, what species of animal provided the blood in question, but the result shows a temperature coefficient of rather less, though not much less, than Hartridge and Roughton(8) found for the sheep by kinetic methods.

There are in addition the experiments of Maçela and Seliškar [9], in which the temperature coefficient of the equilibrium constant in dilute solutions of hæmoglobin was explored. Reference has already been made to these experiments in Chapter v, in which their relation to the problem of specificity is discussed. Here therefore it will only be necessary to treat of them very shortly. The measurements of oxygen content are of course spectroscopic, and in addition there are individual differences between different animals in the same species, both of which factors make the results when plotted appear some-

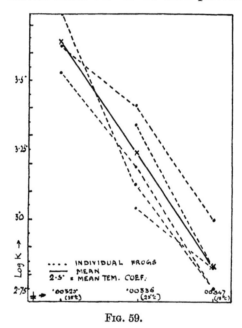

FIG. 59.

what rugged. A good example is that of the blood of the frog. Fig. 59 shows results from the blood of five frogs. The hæmoglobin concentration was made in each case equivalent to one-fortieth of that in normal human blood, i.e. to about a 0·4 per cent. solution. It was buffered to pH = 7·4 and the data are plotted as shown in Fig. 59, the logarithm of the pressure at 50 per cent. saturation forming the ordinate and the reciprocal of the absolute temperature the abscissa. It is quite clear that the temperature coefficient for frog's blood is less than for mammalian blood and it is only about half that of human blood.

Another method of demonstrating that temperature has a great effect on the rate at which oxyhæmoglobin can be reduced is that used by Hill and myself (5). Nitrogen was bubbled through a suitably protected solution of oxyhæmoglobin at a constant rate but at two different temperatures. The rate at which the oxyhæmoglobin was reduced was noted in each case. The experiment was performed thus: We started at a temperature of 18° C. with the blood fully saturated. The course of the experiment may be followed by reference to Figs. 60 and 61—the former shows the apparatus, the latter the results obtained. As regards the apparatus the hæmoglobin solution was

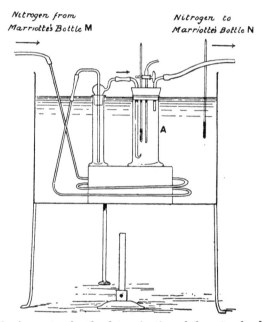

FIG. 60. Apparatus for the determination of the rate of reduction of a hæmoglobin solution.

placed in a cylinder, A. Nitrogen was passed at a constant rate in the direction of the arrows, first through a wash-bottle containing an alkaline solution of pyrogallol, then through the hæmoglobin solution; the whole apparatus was immersed in a water bath in which it was kept at the required temperature. Samples of hæmoglobin, which were small relative to the whole volume of hæmoglobin used, could be abstracted from A at any time through a tube let in through the cork, for the determination of the oxygen saturation. At any time in the experiment the inlet and outlet tubes for the nitrogen could be clamped and the whole apparatus warmed up rapidly by replacing the water in the bath by water at a higher temperature. The flow of nitrogen was then resumed at the altered temperature.

Nitrogen was allowed to run for 35 minutes by which time the hæmoglobin was slightly reduced. An analysis showed that 6 per cent. of the hæmoglobin was reduced hæmoglobin and 94 per cent. was oxyhæmoglobin. The point at which we arrived is represented as *D* on Fig. 61. There is possibly an error of about 2 per cent. in this measurement either way, i.e. the percentage saturation may have been 92 per cent. or 94 per cent. (*d* or *d′*). The nitrogen was stopped, the temperature of the bath was raised to 38° C. (the time taken

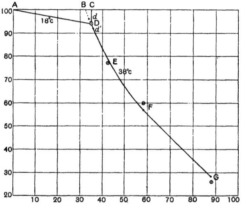

Fig. 61. Curve representing the calculated degree of dissociation, at any time, of hæmoglobin, which was reduced by a stream of nitrogen bubbled at a uniform rate. Percentage saturation plotted vertically, time in minutes horizontally. The points represent actual determinations: *A–D* at 18° C., *D–G* at 38° C.

for the change is omitted from the diagram), and the nitrogen was re-started. The hæmoglobin now became reduced very rapidly. After this three other determinations were made as follows:

Point on curve	D	E	F	G
Time (minutes) measured from *D* ...	0	7·5	23	53
Percentage saturation of hæmoglobin ...	94	77	60	26

Thus, whilst at 18° C., 35 minutes had been required for the reduction of hæmoglobin from 100 to 94 per cent. saturation, at 38° C. it only required 7·5 minutes to reduce it from 94 to 77 per cent. Perhaps the best comparison of the times necessary to produce a given reduction is that obtained by extrapolating the curve *DEFG* backwards to *B*, in which case *AC* represents the time necessary to produce the reduction from 100 to 94 per cent. at 18° C., whilst BC represents the time necessary for the same reduction at 38° C. The former is 35 minutes, the latter is 2·5 or, at most, 3 minutes. Had the alteration in the temperature been not 20° C. but 10° C. the ratio of the times necessary to produce the reduction from 100 to 94 per cent. saturation would have been proportional to the square root of $(35 \div 3)$, i.e. about in the proportion of 3·4 : 1.

The experiments just described were undertaken by Hill and myself with some idea of studying the rates of oxidation and reduction of hæmoglobin in the sense in which Hartridge and Roughton have carried out the work. Everything that we know, however, suggests that the rate of reduction of the hæmoglobin was controlled not by

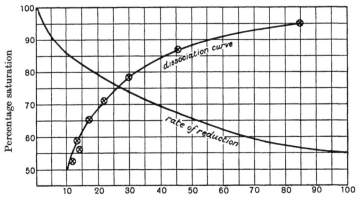

FIG. 62. Abscissa for rate of reduction = minutes; for dissociation curve = arbitrary unit of pressure.

the velocity constant of the reduction process, but by the rate of diffusion of oxygen from the fluid into the bubble. What took place is conceived as being somewhat as follows. The pressure of oxygen in the fluid at any moment was that which corresponds, on the oxygen dissociation curve, to the percentage saturation of the hæmoglobin at that moment—call this pressure p. The pressure of oxygen in the bubble was nil, for only a negligible amount of oxygen diffused into any one bubble. The rate of diffusion of oxygen from the fluid at any saturation then was proportional to $p - 0$, i.e. to p.

If that is so it should be possible to reconstruct the dissociation curve in shape, i.e. to plot the percentage saturation against something which is proportional to the pressure. This calculation was attempted with the data given in the two experiments in Barcroft and Hill's paper; the data, however, are not available below 50 per cent. saturation. Down to that point Fig. 62 shows (a) a dissociation curve calculated from Hill's equation ($n = 1\cdot32$), (b) points calculated from the data given in the second experiment of Barcroft and Hill. It will be seen that the points fall on a reasonable dissociation curve for the hæmoglobin.

From the other curve of reduction given in the paper (5) a dissociation curve can be extracted of much the same type as that in Fig. 62. It would be interesting to repeat and see whether the dissociation curve of the solution determined by the bubbling method agreed with that actually found by the normal method of equilibration.

The above results; however, seem to show that the increase in the rate of reduction on the rise of temperature is in fact ruled by the temperature coefficient of the oxygen dissociation curve, which would appear therefore to be between 3 and 4.

The effect of rise of temperature, then, is to drive oxygen out of hæmoglobin, other things being equal; that statement carries with it by implication another, namely, that when oxygen is driven out of hæmoglobin heat is absorbed, or to put it the other way, when oxygen unites with hæmoglobin heat is given out. It is naturally a matter of some interest to determine the amount of heat given out when a molecule of oxygen unites with an equivalent of hæmoglobin. This may be determined experimentally, it may also be calculated from the oxygen dissociation curve. It seems better first to consider the latter method because the reader will see what opportunities there are for a want of uniformity in the final answer. The fact is, as will appear later, that different workers have found very different values for the heat of formation of oxyhæmoglobin, and in considering them it is as well to be aware of the extent to which a want of uniformity may reasonably be looked for. Therefore, to take the matter up thermodynamically (if I may use so resonant a word to describe any process of treatment to be found in these pages), conceive of a solution of hæmoglobin in equilibrium with oxygen and, say, 64 per cent. saturated at a certain temperature, say 26° C., the oxygen pressure is, according to Fig. 57, 12·5 mm.; now gradually raise the temperature; in order to prevent the saturation falling the oxygen pressure must be raised also, and at 38° C. the pressure will be 31 mm. The heat of combination (Q) of one molecule of oxygen at that particular percentage saturation is found as follows:

$$Q = 2\cdot303 \times R \times \frac{T_1 T_2}{T_1 - T_2} \times \log \frac{p_2}{p_1},$$

where T_1 and T_2 are the initial and final absolute temperatures, in this case 299° and 311° C., and p_1 and p_2 are the pressures at which the hæmoglobin is 64 per cent. saturated at those temperatures.

In the nature of things, as has already been said, Q need not be the same for all saturations, but so far as the present experimental evidence goes Q is the same for all saturations on the same sample of hæmoglobin because the ratio of p_2 to p_1 seems to be the same right up the curve. Therefore, in theory, the same amount of heat should be given out per 32 grams of oxygen absorbed, whether that oxygen is employed partially or completely saturating the hæmoglobin. In actual practice some observers of the heat developed have adopted the method of partial and others complete oxidation; the answer should come out the same and therefore it is open to the experimenter to use whichever method offers fewest opportunities of experimental error, but remembering that the validity of what he is doing depends upon the constancy of the ratio of p_2/p_1 for any given saturation at two different temperatures.

The next point which perhaps may be taken up is the shape of the curves. Clearly different samples of hæmoglobin give curves of different shapes: one may give a nearly hyperbolic curve, another a curve which is considerably inflected. An example may be found in my own work published with Hill. On two occasions we subjected a hæmoglobin solution to a given pressure of oxygen at different temperatures, noted the saturations, assumed the hyperbolic nature of the curve and then made a calculation which in essence amounted to finding the pressures at which the hæmoglobin was 50 per cent. saturated at the various temperatures (or indeed saturated to any other given point). Where do those calculations stand if the curve is not a hyperbola? As a matter of fact two of the temperatures in question are the same as those used by King and myself, two others are so close that a comparison can easily be made. Thus:

(1)	Temperature (° C.)	16	25	32	38	—
	Observed saturations ...	96	89	77	52	—
	Saturations at 22 mm. (Barcroft and King's curves) ...	98	89·5	75·5	52	—
(2)	Temperature (° C.)	16	24	32	38	49
	Observed saturations ...	90	71	41	22	6
	Saturations at 11·5 mm. (Barcroft and King's curves) ...	95	69	41	22	—

Granting then that the data fit well enough to be applied to these curves, we may proceed to calculate the heat of formation of hæmoglobin from the curves and to compare it with values obtained from hyperbolic curves.

Applying the data given above, namely, that at 64 per cent. saturation the oxygen pressure at $26°$ C. is $12·5$ mm. and at $38°$ C. it is 31 mm., the value of Q comes out to be 14,000 calories. The value given by the "hyperbolic" calculation brought it out at 27,700. If, however, our experimental technique had consisted not in measuring percentage saturations at a given pressure but pressures at a given percentage saturation (something in practice much more difficult), our calculation of Q would have been unaffected by the degree of inflection of the curve. It should here be made very clear that Q is the heat evolved when one *molecule of oxygen* unites with hæmoglobin, it makes no assumption as to the number of molecules of oxygen which unite with one molecule of hæmoglobin, nor is it a matter of any interest now from that point of view for the molecular weight of hæmoglobin has been determined in other ways.

If 32 grams or $22·4$ litres of oxygen give out 14,000 calories it remains to calculate the quantity of heat given out by $1·34$ c.c. of oxygen when it unites with 1 gram of hæmoglobin. That comes out to $·85$ calorie, and the question must then be asked: How does that figure compare with the experimental data?

Many observers have determined experimentally the heat evolved when hæmoglobin unites with oxygen, and have arrived at very varying results. Putting aside observations which have been made upon blood, and considering only observations made on hæmoglobin, the following data are collected by Adolf and Henderson [10]:

Author	Heat in calories per gram of Hb oxidised			
	Number of observations	Extreme limits (max.)	Extreme limits (min.)	Animal
Torup [11]	4	0·75	0·62	Horse
Barcroft and Hill [5] ...	3	1·98	1·62	Dog
Du Bois Raymond [12] ...	4	1·14	0·8	Horse
Adolf and Henderson [10] ...	—	0·66	0·09	—

From the above data I learn that I enjoy the distinction of having obtained a figure higher than that of any other observer—a circumstance which reminds me of the novel in which it is recorded of the hero—"no one in the boat that day rowed a faster stroke than bow"—I quote from memory.

But, seriously, what is to be said of such discrepancies? Adolf and Henderson after pointing out in this connection what a very complex affair is the oxidation of hæmoglobin, say:

In the light of these considerations it is perhaps not surprising that simple theory and complex fact are apparently at variance. The discrepancies may be summarised for the present in the statement that the active mass of hæmoglobin differs in its measurable properties in its behaviour towards oxygen.

Perhaps, but it goes a little against the grain to leave the matter there, and I should not be surprised if one day my curiosity will drive me to explore, if possible, the reason why Hill and I obtained so high a result. If I was asked to pick out the researches in my past, in the purely experimental measurements of which I had least confidence, that particular research would not be among them.

It only remains to be said that several workers have made estimates of the heat evolved when carbon monoxide unites with hæmoglobin; it is a little but only a little higher than when oxygen takes part in the parallel reaction. The result is that the reaction, the displacement of oxygen by CO from oxyhæmoglobin, is accompanied by an evolution of heat which, according to Adolf and Henderson, is only about one-fifth of that involved in the union of CO with reduced hæmoglobin; the latter, according to them, being 15,000 calories per molecule of COHb formed, the former about 3000 calories per molecule of oxygen displaced by CO. The results obtained on CO-hæmoglobin are more uniform than those obtained on hæmoglobin, but even they vary in the case of Adolf and Henderson's experiments from 11,000 to 28,000 calories.

REFERENCES

(1) BARCROFT AND KING. *Journ. Physiol.* XXXIX. 374. 1909.

(2) BERT, PAUL. *La Pression Barométrique.* Paris, 1878.

(3) HÜFNER. *Zeitsch. f. Physiol. Chem.* XII and XIII. 1889.

(4) BROWN AND HILL. *Proc. Roy. Soc.* B. XCIV. 297. 1923.

(5) BARCROFT AND HILL. *Journ. Physiol.* XXXIX. 411. 1910.

(6) BOHR, CHR. *Zentralb. f. Physiol.* V. 187. 1901.

(7) HENDERSON, L. J. *Journ. Biol. Chem.* XLI. 401. 1920.

(8) HARTRIDGE AND ROUGHTON. *Proc. Roy. Soc.* A. CIV. 395. 1923.

(9) MAÇELA AND SELIŠKAR. *Journ. Physiol.* LX. 428. 1925.

(10) ADOLF AND HENDERSON, L. J. *Journ. Biol. Chem.* L. 463. 1922.
    [Contains an excellent bibliography of the subject.]

(11) TORUP. (Quoted from *Festschrift für Olof Hammersten.* 1906.)

(12) DU BOIS RAYMOND. *Arch. f. Anat. u. Physiol.* p. 237. 1914.

CHAPTER XVII

THE BIOLOGICAL SIGNIFICANCE OF HÆMOGLOBIN

THE question which always recurs is: What is hæmoglobin? It may be asked from the chemical or the biological standpoint—one commences with the chemical aspect, one concludes with the biological. Hæmoglobin, biologically, possesses the following properties:

(1) It is capable of transporting a large quantity of oxygen from one place to another. This it might be supposed to do either because a small amount of hæmoglobin could attach itself to a large amount of oxygen, or because a large hæmoglobin molecule can unite with a relatively small oxygen molecule. The latter alternative, which is the one actually in existence, demands that hæmoglobin should be very soluble, we therefore come to the second important property of hæmoglobin, namely,

(2) Great solubility.

(3) Hæmoglobin must unite with oxygen at a suitable velocity and in sufficient amount under the circumstances in which it finds itself in the blood, and must give it up in proper quantities under the circumstances which prevail in the tissues. This interaction is facilitated by the fourth important property of hæmoglobin, namely, that

(4) Carbonic acid tends to expel oxygen from hæmoglobin and, conversely, oxygen tends to expel carbonic acid from alkaline solutions which contain that gas.

Let us turn now to see if we can trace some of the steps by which a material with these remarkable properties has been produced.

Of these the first is the fact of its forming a reversible compound with oxygen. If one goes back to the simpler compounds from which hæmoglobin may be regarded as being synthesised, none of them has this property. The facts which stand out are that hæmatin and its compounds are capable of oxidation and reduction, but that in order to effect the reduction a chemical reducer is always necessary. These substances then would be useless for a system such as prevails in the body, in which the oxygen carrier is circulated in a blood-vessel, whilst the actual oxidation takes place in a tissue situated at a little distance. Over this distance the oxygen must travel as molecular oxygen. What then is the determining factor? Evidently it is in some way associated with the protein portion of the hæmoglobin molecule. But even when the issue has been narrowed to the protein portion, the precise cause of the reversibility of the reaction with oxygen is remarkable; hæmatin forms many compounds with protein, and many compounds with bodies similar to protein, but it is only compounds with one class of protein bodies—the globins—which can behave in this way. Indeed we can narrow the issue still further, for the compounds of hæmatin and denatured globin do not form reversible compounds with oxygen; nor does methæmoglobin, which differs from hæmoglobin by containing iron in the ferric state (Conant). The essential point, however, is that the globin compound of hæmatin possesses the power of undergoing the transformation necessary to effect the lability of the oxygen—no other compounds of hæmatin do so.

Not that the analogues of hæmochromogen are insufficiently numerous. Many nitrogenous substances exist with which hæmatin makes compounds on the hæmochromogen level, but Robin Hill was unable to make a hæmoglobin analogue out of any but the globin compound, though he has tried quite a number.

Why the oxygen in hæmoglobin should be easily dissociated whilst that in hæmochromogen is not, remains for the present, a mystery. A further mystery is furnished by the fact that the general analogy between the oxygen and carbon monoxide compounds of hæmoglobin breaks down at this point. Carbon monoxide dissociates from hæmoglobin much less readily than oxygen, nevertheless CO forms a compound with hæmochromogen that breaks down in the presence of a CO vacuum whilst the oxygen compound does not. That at least is the way in which the matter is presented in the literature, but we do not know really what the "CO compound of hæmochromogen" is. It was assumed by Anson and Mirsky to be a body made by the addition of CO to hæmochromogen. In that case it seems to bear no real analogy to anything which is formed on the oxidation of hæmochromogen, for this latter reaction appears to be associated with the splitting of the hæmatin from the globin. It may be that CO can combine with the $C_{34}H_{30}O_4N_4FeOH$ without tearing it away from the globin, and it may be that this is the reason why the CO compound is reversible—we do not know. Here we must be content simply to confess our ignorance, and point out that before we have a complete understanding of hæmoglobin we must discover why globin, of all things, is the only substance which is capable of forming a compound with reduced hæmatin, which has the significant property of hæmoglobin, to wit, the possibility of a dissociable oxygen compound.

Until recently one had supposed that the great "find" which nature had made was hæmatin, whilst it was a matter of quite secondary importance that the hæmatin had been united to a protein, but no one suggested that it was a matter of any particular importance what protein was involved. I will not say that the tables are now turned, because hæmatin does seem to be very much better for its purpose than anything else, but one must point out the difference between hæmoglobin and chlorocruorin, another iron-containing pigment which is analogous to hæmoglobin. This pigment is found in certain worms and was first studied by Ray Lankester; lately it has been the subject of extended research by H. Munro Fox.

Chlorocruorin has a complete set of derivatives (to use the hackneyed phrase, which seems to infer a logical precedence of the cart to the horse); it has compounds analogous to hæmatin, to hæmochromogen, and presumably the relation of chlorocruorin to chlorocruorochromogen is the same as that of hæmoglobin to hæmochromogen, and in each case the change accounts in the same way for the dissociability of the oxygen. So far as I know the protein moiety has not been investigated, but presumably it is a globin.

The essential difference between chlorocruorin and hæmoglobin is to be found in the hæmatin from which the chromogen is derived. In each case the hæmatin is an iron-containing compound, and in each case the iron may be split off leaving a porphyrin, but the two porphyrins are different. The point I wish to emphasise is that this difference in the porphyrins only affects the molecules quantitatively. Qualitatively their properties are the same. It is probable that this quantitative difference is enough to make chlorocruorin unsuited to the needs of mammalian metabolism, so chlorocruorin has, as it were, dropped out of the hunt; the difference in the porphyrins is insufficient to upset the whole properties of the molecule.

But one may go further and dispense with the iron altogether without essentially changing the molecular character. Hæmocyanin possesses the same general properties as hæmoglobin, but in a very restricted degree; for which reason the molluscs, in so far as they preferred hæmocyanin to hæmoglobin, took a course which confined their development to the level of the octopus.

When I say that the molluscs preferred hæmocyanin to hæmoglobin, naturally I am using no more than a figure of speech. It is, of course, not my meaning that in the evolution of the snail any conscious selection of pigments was made, yet the figure of speech stands for a very striking phenomenon—a phenomenon as striking as if a deliberate choice had been made and the die cast in favour of the copper compound. For in some snails you get the copper and iron compounds side by side. The hæmocyanin is the respiratory pigment found in the blood-vessels; the helicorubin, which is a hæmochromogen, is thrust from the liver into the alimentary canal. Why it is not the other way round we do not know. Why is not the copper pigment thrust out and the iron one retained and circulated as hæmoglobin in the blood-vessels? Here again we do not know. Whatever may be the cause, it appears that there is no case in which hæmoglobin is found in the presence of hæmocyanin, though it is not unknown for hæmocyanin to be found in the presence of the hæmochromogen. And it may be that the protein of helicorubin is too far removed from globin to make the formation of hæmoglobin from helicorubin possible; at least the spectroscopic evidence rather lends itself to that reading of the situation. We shall see in a moment that there are a great many different hæmoglobins, the difference being, as far as we can tell, in the globins; yet all these globins are so nearly alike that the spectra of the hæmochromogens derived from them are indistinguishable. Not merely are they of the same type but the positions of the bands are the same within the limits of the error of reading. The spectrum of helicorubin is a hæmochromogen spectrum, inasmuch as it is of the hæmochromogen type, but it could be distinguished from globin-hæmochromogen by a difference in position of the bands.

When we come to the hæmochromogens we find that the field over which we have to look is as broad as it was narrow in the case of hæmoglobin. Of these the one which claims our attention in the first instance is cytochrome. Cytochrome has been so fully dealt with at the commencement of this book that here it is only necessary to recall the fact of its almost universal distribution over the animal kingdom, of its apparent function as a catalyst, and of its being a hæmochromogen, if not a group of hæmochromogens.

When one tries to get behind the hæmochromogens, to find out, as it were, what is their ancestry, one is at present in the dim ages of chemical evolution. One looks in several directions—Are there simpler bodies of the conjugated protein type? or again, if one takes the two moieties of the conjugated protein—Are there bodies from which one can suppose that they have been derived? Along the line of the protein we are lost at once. I suppose there is no form of animal life but contains some protein to which $C_{34}H_{30}O_4N_4FeOH$ might not conceivably attach itself. Along the line of the pigment we have to consider what substances may have been the precursors of $C_{34}H_{30}O_4N_4FeOH$.

There has not lacked speculation on this subject, and a number of obvious materials present themselves for our consideration. Of these mention may first be made of the porphyrins. It is a commonplace that a large literature has grown up around these substances within the last few years. At present one can only say that there are quite a number of cases which might be cited in which porphyrins occur in animal tissues—the dorsal line on the back of the earthworm, the pigment of the hen's egg-shell, and the pigment laid down in the bones and teeth of cases of hæmatoporphyrinuria; to say nothing of the kindred bile pigments; but it cannot be said of any of these that they are a stage on the up-grade to hæmoglobin, or indeed that they are ever made in the body out of anything but hæmoglobin. Certainly bile pigments and the pigment of the egg-shell are degradation products; of the other two cases cited we know nothing one way or the other. It has been pointed out to me by Sir Frederick Hopkins, that an attractive analogy might be drawn between porphyrinuria and other complaints, such as cystinuria and alcaptanuria, and that these substances appear to be produced as the result of the stoppage of a synthetic process; but this is at best only an analogy, and it has not been suggested that the analogy could be driven home.

The porphyrins are of two main classes. It is a little remarkable that hæmatoporphyrin, the form of porphyrin which is obtained in hæmatoporphyrinuria, is not that which might be expected to occur as a stage in the formation of hæmoglobin: that would be protoporphyrin, the form found in the egg-shell is a direct derivative of hæmoglobin.

In our discussion we have left over the finer points of the globin influence. At the point at which we left the matter we had said that the globins in the various hæmochromogens of which hæmoglobin is made were so nearly the same that spectroscopically they cannot be separated. Nevertheless different hæmoglobins differ greatly. It is rather for future research to discover the precise biological significance of these differences. It is not suggested for instance that it is a matter of any moment what crystalline form a particular hæmoglobin assumes. That is not to say that the factor in the molecule which decides the crystalline form may not be very important for other reasons. I only wish to warn the reader lest he should think that because he discovers a fact, that fact may have a biological significance, and I take crystalline form as an example, because so far as I know hæmoglobin in a functional state never occurs in crystals, and therefore the form in which it crystallises is of no importance. It is when we come to the relationship of hæmoglobin to gases that we have to consider rather closely whether such facts as we observe are biologically significant. It seems quite clear that different forms of life are possessed of hæmoglobins with fundamentally different affinities for oxygen. For instance, man, *Planorbis* and the frog at 15° C. have very different dissociation curves —that is an understatement, man and the frog have affinities of quite a different order at 15° C. Has this fact any biological significance? The first point that occurs to me is that human hæmoglobin does not operate at 15° C. but at 37° C. or thereabouts. But at what temperature does frog's hæmoglobin function? It may operate at 37° C. in the swamps of tropical Florida, or at 7° C. in the ponds during the British frosty spring time, and therefore not only must its properties be appropriate to some one temperature, but the temperature coefficient of its affinity to oxygen must be such as to adapt it to the uses of the body over a wide range, and therefore cannot be quite a haphazard affair—it must be related to the temperature coefficients of other chemical processes in the frog. In the case of man one may speculate too upon whether the temperature coefficient has any particular meaning. It appears to be more than twice that of the frog, and instead of being about 2 it is somewhere in the region of 5.

Now it may be that in an organism so nearly homoiothermic as man it is a matter of no importance whether hæmoglobin has any temperature coefficient at all, but if the temperature coefficient is to be of importance, clearly it must be very high. If, for instance, it is important that during exercise or fever hæmoglobin should dissociate from oxygen more rapidly than at normal body temperature, a small temperature coefficient would effect nothing. On the other hand, the high temperature coefficient of human hæmoglobin may be just an accident, it may be abnormal just because it does not matter and there is nothing to make it matter. In that case it comes to be as it is because the particular globin with which the hæmatin is united is not of significance from the point of view of temperature.

So much then for the fact that hæmoglobin transports oxygen. It remains to be said that the equivalent of about 17,000 grams transports only 32 grams of oxygen and therefore great solubility is required. Here again we find that the solubility is conferred on the iron-containing hæmatin—a very insoluble substance—by the protein, and that among proteins globin is far the most efficient, so that globin performs the double function of rendering the oxygen labile and the molecule soluble.

We now come to the third of the fundamental properties with which this discussion was started, namely, that the pressures at which the oxygen is acquired and given up should be such that the oxidation of the hæmoglobin is as nearly as possible complete in the lung and its reduction easy in the capillaries of the tissues. Krogh has introduced a nomenclature to express the point numerically. He calls the partial pressure of oxygen to which the hæmoglobin is exposed in the lung or gill "the tension of loading," and that at which the hæmoglobin becomes 50 per cent. reduced "the tension of unloading." With this nomenclature at our service let us review the position. When considering the temperature coefficients we assumed the hæmoglobin to be in the fundamental condition in which such things must be considered if a start is to be made in the investigation of their properties, namely, in a dilute solution under some sort of standard circumstances. The evidence on the subject is not beyond reproach, but at present it seems to point to the dissociation curve being a hyperbola under such fundamental circumstances. This, if true, is of great interest, firstly, because a curve of that shape is extremely ill-suited to the needs of the intensive form of respiration which alone makes the warm-blooded animal as we know it possible, and secondly, because the hyperbolic curve forms a simple starting-point from which we may hope to derive the more complicated curves that are actually found in the body. Not only may we hope to derive these curves but we may hope also to discern the process of evolution which nature has fixed upon in order to obtain a curve suitable to her purpose.

Firstly, then, as regards the most suitable combinations of tensions for loading and unloading. It is clear that the tension of loading cannot be higher than that of the oxygen in atmospheric air—unless, indeed, some secretion process is at work in the lung; and of course there are reasons why it should be lower. In the lung of the warm-blooded animal there must be upwards of 50 mm. pressure of aqueous vapour and a considerable amount of CO_2, and the fact that the lung is an almost closed bag from which oxygen is always being abstracted means a considerable reduction in the pressure of the oxygen to which the blood is exposed. Thus the tension of loading comes to be in the vicinity of 100 mm. of mercury. That of unloading is about 40 mm. Obviously it is desirable that the tension of unloading should be sufficiently high in order to provide a pressure head capable of effecting the passage of considerable quantities of gas from the capillary to the tissue at the moments when the metabolism of the tissue is most intense.

In human blood the pressures of oxygen in the blood of the right and left sides of the heart respectively are approximately 40 and 100 mm., the saturations about 66 and 96 per cent. That is to say the blood can lose about 30 per cent. of its oxygen, at so high a pressure as 40 mm., which pressure is the driving force available for the expulsion of the oxygen from the capillaries into the tissues.

If the dissociation curve were a hyperbola how much oxygen would hæmoglobin part with between the pressures of 100 and 40 mm.? To answer the question we may consider two hyperbolæ, one of which, like arterial blood, is 96 per cent. saturated at 100 mm. pressure, the other, like venous blood, is 66 per cent. saturated at 40 mm. pressure.

The hyperbola which indicates 96 per cent. saturation at 100 mm. would indicate about 91 per cent. saturation at 40 mm., and so the hæmoglobin would only have lost 5–6 per cent. of its oxygen in the transition. On the other hand, the hyperbola which yields 66 per cent. saturation at 40 mm. will only indicate 83 per cent. saturation at 100 mm. so that there will only be a gain or loss of 17 per cent. in the circuit. In either case the system would be very inefficient: in the latter five-sixths of the hæmoglobin is being carried round the body to no purpose, in the former nineteen-twentieths. Hæmoglobin depends for its biological efficiency upon the double inflection of its curve; that property it shares with hæmocyanin—a quite different substance, containing not iron but copper, and containing no porphyrin, but which is like hæmoglobin a conjugated protein; but hæmoglobin does not share this double inflection with its neighbour hæmochromogen, from which it differs only in the matter of the

protein, CO-hæmochromogen has a hyperbolic dissociation curve.
It would seem therefore that the double inflection was in some way a
function of the protein, but how? Well, the reader may read Chapter XII
once more and may see whether he there finds a really satisfactory
answer to the question. If not he has food enough for thought. Sometimes I have wondered whether the double inflection depended upon
some question of solubility, but no simple combination of a hyperbola
with a dissociation curve, such as shown in Fig. 63, will meet the case.

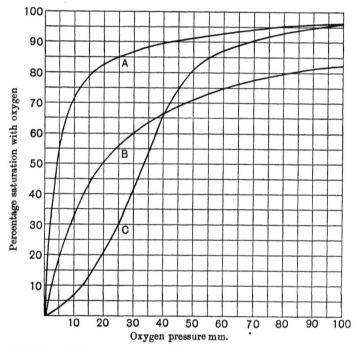

FIG. 63. A. Hyperbola corresponding to 96 per cent. saturation and 100 mm. pressure.
B. Hyperbola corresponding to 40 per cent. saturation and 66·6 mm. pressure.
C. Dissociation curve of blood (Christiansen, Douglas and Haldane).

Not only is the dissociation curve of blood wonderfully efficient
in view of the considerations which have just been stated, but almost
as interesting is its reserve capacity. Every form of life must
face emergencies and the one which survives them is that best
calculated to meet the strain. Now here the necessary form of adjustment, or one factor in it, is that when the tissue requires a greater
supply of oxygen the blood should be capable of imparting it with

the least possible drop in the pressure at which it leaves. Look then! with the loss of another 10 mm. pressure the blood curve imparts another 25 per cent. of all its oxygen, the hæmoglobin curves 4–6 per cent.

And we come to the last of the four properties which, at the commencement of this chapter, I set forth as giving hæmoglobin its great biological significance, namely, its power of buffering a bicarbonate solution and thus of enabling the body to deal with the production of large quantities of carbonic acid without the CO_2 produced setting up great changes of hydrogen-ion concentration in the blood, and also without its causing so great a rise of CO_2-pressure in blood as to dam the gas back in the tissues. About this we know more. After a battle as to whether the buffering property of hæmoglobin is due to its own power of uniting with carbonic acid or simply to its acting itself as an acid in competition with CO_2 and claiming the bicarbonate, opinion has set itself firmly in favour of the latter view. But the buffering power of hæmoglobin is not merely due to its composition; it is due in part to the fact of its being housed in corpuscles. The red corpuscle and its properties must form the subject of the other volume, and so of this the end.

INDEX

acid hæmatin, 17

action of CO_2, 188

Adair, 67, 70, 78, 79, 80, 81, 99, 108, 110, 115, 126, 129 *et seq.*, 177

Adam, K. Neil, 120

Adolf, 99, 186, 187

adsorption hypothesis, 52, 58, 118

affinity of CO, 3

aggregation, 75

albumin hæmochromogen, 20

alcaptanuria, 192

alcohol, action on cytochrome, 35; use of, 64, 65, 66

aldehyde, action on cytochrome, 35

aluminium porphyrin, 14

ammonia hæmochromogen, 20

Anson, 2, 3, 19 *et seq.*, 102, 189

Arenicola, 41, 45, 47

Arnold, 61

Arrhenius' equation, 145

baboon, hæmoglobin of, 39, 40

Bacillus subtilis, cytochrome in, 30, 36

Balfour, F. M., 7, 13

Barcroft, J., 66, 67, 70, 131, 156, 181, 185, 186

base-free hæmoglobin, 82

bat, hæmoglobin of, 40

Bayliss, W. M., 58, 60, 72

bee's muscle, cytochrome in, 26, 30, 31

benzidine, 37

Bert, Paul, 175

Bertin-Sans and Moitessier, 18

biological significance of hæmoglobin, 188

birds, cytochrome in, 36

Blackwood, Algernon, 72

blow-fly, cytochrome in, 32

Bock, 103

Bohr, Christian, 54, 60, 65, 67, 97, 111, 148, 151

Bohr's theory, 123

Brown, A. S., *see* Reichert

Brown, W. E. L., 175

buffering action of hæmoglobin, 113, 117

Butterfield, 54

calibration of differential apparatus, 58

Camis, 174

carbon monoxide, 3; effect on moths, 4; effect on seedlings, 4

carbonic acid on dissociation curve, 110

carboxyhæmoglobin, 47, 48, 49, 148, 161

carp, hæmoglobin of, 41

catalytic properties of cytochrome, 35

centrifuge, Svedberg's, 89

chemical relation between Hb and O_2, 178

Chironomus, 41, 43

chlorocruorin, 12, 13, 190

chloroform action on cytochrome, 35

chlorophyll, 1, 2, 7, 37

Church, 14

CO_2, use in manufacture of Hb, 67

cobalt porphyrin, 14

cockroach, cytochrome of, 80

CO-hæmochromogen, 3

colloid on turacin, 16

Conant, 52, 189

Conant's theory, 122

concentration of hæmoglobin, measurement of, 78

copper porphyrin, 14

coproporphyrin, 7, 11

corpuscle, condition of hæmoglobin in, 5

crystals of hæmoglobin, 1, 38

cystinuria, 192

cytochrome, 2, 26 *et seq.*; function of, 34; in *Dytiscus*, 30; in frog, 30, 36; in *Galleria*, 30; in snail, 30, 31, 36

Derrien, 7

Dhéré, 7

dialysed hæmoglobin, 66, 99

differential blood gas apparatus, 58

Dilling, 18

dog, hæmoglobin of, 39, 42, 48, 49, 63, 65, 67

Douglas, 1, 44, 105, 111, 123, 126, 148, 151, 168

Dudley, 66

earthworm, porphyrin in, 7

Edkins, 99

egg-shell, porphyrin in, 7

electrolytes, 9

equation, Hill's, 105

equilibrium, between CO, O_2, and Hb, 161, 164; constant effect of temperature on, 177

Eschalot, cytochrome in, 30

ether, use of, 64, 65, 66

Euonymus, 37

Evans, 66

ferricyanide method, 54

Ferry, 39, 99

Fischer, Hans, 7 *et seq.*

flour, hæmatin in, 33

Forbes, 43, 157

Foster, Sir Michael, 1, 7

fowl, 41, 48, 49

fox, hæmoglobin of, 39

Fox, H. Munro, 3, 12, 190

freezing point, depression of, 87

frog, hæmoglobin of, 44, 46, 49, 193